汉英对照口袋书(彩图版)
Chinese-English Pocket Edition (Colored)

足部反射区按摩图解
Illustrations of Foot Reflex Zone Massage

主　编　王亚渭
主　译　李永安　张　焱
译　者　曲倩倩　董　娜
　　　　王　萱　王　丹

Chief Editor　Wang Ya-wei
Chief Translators　Li Yong-an　Zhang Yan
Translators　Qu Qian-qian　Dong Na
　　　　　　　Wang Xuan　Wang Dan

上海科学技术出版社
Shanghai Scientific and Technical Publishers

图书在版编目(CIP)数据

足部反射区按摩图解:汉英对照/王亚渭主编;李永安,张焱主译.—上海:上海科学技术出版社,2009.10
(汉英对照口袋书:彩图版)
ISBN 978-7-5323-9644-3

Ⅰ.足… Ⅱ.①王…②李…③张… Ⅲ.足-按摩疗法(中医)-图解 Ⅳ.R244.1-64

中国版本图书馆 CIP 数据核字(2008)第 178045 号

上海世纪出版股份有限公司
上海 科 学 技 术 出 版 社 出版发行
(上海钦州南路71号 邮政编码200235)
新华书店上海发行所经销
浙江新华印刷技术有限公司印刷
开本 889×1194 1/64 印张 2.75
字数 126千字
2009年10月第1版 2009年10月第1次印刷
ISBN 978-7-5323-9644-3/R·2595
定价:30.00元

本书如有缺页、错装或坏损等严重质量问题,请向工厂联系调换

内容提要

本书为"汉英对照口袋书(彩图版)"丛书之一分册。全书分四章阐述了足部反射区按摩的起源和发展、概念、作用以及与其他疗法的关系,入门要领和医学原理;详细介绍了足部反射区定位和操作,配有161张彩色照片,并介绍了双足整体按摩在临床的应用。全书图文并茂、通俗易懂、汉英对照,可供广大海内外足部反射区按摩医师和爱好者学习、参考。

Synopsis

This book is one of the volumes of series of *Chinese-English Pocket Edition (Colored) Illustrations*. The book contains four chapters which expounds the foot reflex zone massage in terms of the origin, development, conception, function, its relations with other therapies, rudimentary essentials, and medical principles. It also elaborates the location and the operation of foot reflex zones, along with 161 colored photographs. In addition, the book introduces the clinical application of the integral massage of both feet. The whole book features text with pictures, easy-to-read style, and Chinese-English layout, which is suitable for domestic and overseas foot reflex zone massage doctors and enthusiasts to learn and consult.

目录

第一章 绪言 ——————————————— 2
  第一节 足部反射区按摩的起源与发展 /2
  第二节 足部反射区按摩的概念、作用以及与其他疗法的关系 /6
  第三节 足部反射区按摩的入门要领 /10

第二章 足部反射区按摩的医学原理 ——————— 16
  第一节 阴阳平衡理论 /16
  第二节 神经反射学说 /18
  第三节 血液循环原理 /18
  第四节 经络学说 /20
  第五节 生物全息论学说 /22
  第六节 心理作用 /22

第三章 足部反射区定位和操作 ———————— 26
  第一节 足部反射区大体定位与对应关系以及按摩手法 /26
  第二节 足部反射区具体定位、操作及适应证 /44

第四章 双足整体按摩 ——————————— 150
  第一节 基本反射区 /150
  第二节 直接反射区 /150
  第三节 相关反射区 /152
  第四节 配区结合原则 /154

Contents

Chapter 1 Introduction —————————————— 3
    Section 1   The Origin and Development of Foot Reflex Zone Massage /3
    Section 2   Foot Reflex Zone Massage: Conception, Functions, and its Relations with Other Therapies /7
    Section 3   The Rudimentary Essentials of Foot Reflex Zone Massage /11

Chapter 2 The Medical Principles of Foot Reflex Zone Massage —————————————— 17
    Section 1   The Theory of Balance between Yin and Yang /17
    Section 2   The Doctrine of Nervous Reflex /19
    Section 3   The Principle of Blood Circulation /19
    Section 4   The Theory of Meridians and Collaterals /21
    Section 5   The Doctrine of Biological Hologram /23
    Section 6   Psychological Effect /23

Chapter 3 Location and Operation of Foot Reflex Zones —————————————— 27
    Section 1   Foot Reflex Zones: Rough Location, Corresponding relations and Manipulations of Massage /27

Section 2 Foot Reflex Zones: Specific Location, Performance and Indications /45

Chapter 4 Integral Massage of Two Feet —————151

  Section 1 Basic Reflex Zones /151
  Section 2 Direct Reflex Zones /151
  Section 3 Correlated Reflex Zones /153
  Section 4 The Principles of Allocation and Combination of Reflex Zones /155

第一章 绪 言

第一节 足部反射区按摩的起源与发展

【起源】

从医学的发展史来看,按摩治病,远远早于应用工具、草药或其他医疗方法。古代足部按摩的形成与跳舞有一定的关系,古人类在地上赤脚跳舞时到足底部发热、舒服,既解除疲劳又振奋精神,当有病痛的人感觉自己的病痛有所缓解后,就加以总结。这是足部按摩的启蒙阶段。先秦时期,在《史记·扁鹊仓公列传》中记载的"俞跗"从名字的字意上推断可能是以按摩足部治病的人。东汉时期的名医华佗发明的"五禽戏"也很重视足部导引。

4500年前在埃及金字塔中有一幅奴隶为巴路王按摩脚的图,上面还有一问一答的对话。古代印度也有关于足部按摩的史证,前释迦人留下了佛都的"佛足石",在这个足印上就有人体与足部相关联的图,古印度的瑜伽术乃受此影响而产生。

Chapter 1 Introduction
Section 1 The Origin and Development of Foot Reflex Zone Massage

Origin

From the historical development of medical science, massage applied to cure diseases had arisen far earlier than tools, medicinal herbs and other therapies. In ancient times, the foot massage had something to do with dancing. The ancient people used to dance barefoot on the ground. When they danced until they felt hot in soles and comfortable, they became refreshed with fatigue relieved. When people with ailment felt their pains somewhat soothed, they began to summarize it. Hence appeared the commencement stage of foot massage. *Shi Ji·Bian Que Cang Gong Lie Zhuan (Memoirs of Bian Que Cang Gong, Records of the Grand Historian)* records the legend of Yu Fu, who lived in the period before the Qin Dynasty. Being inferred from the literal meaning of the name, "Yu Fu" supposedly refers to a person who practiced foot massage to cure diseases. In the Eastern Han Dynasty, the renowned doctor Hua Tuo devised Wuqinxi (Frolics of the Five Animals) which attaches great importance to foot daoyin (leading).

About 4,500 years ago, there was a mural depicting a slave massaging feet for the Pharaoh Baru in an Egyptian Pyramid. The picture also included a conversation with questions and answers. In ancient India, there was also historical evidence about foot massage. For instance, pre-Sakya people handed down the "Buddha's Footprint Stone" from the capital city of Buddha. On the footprints there are pictures of interrelations between human body and feet. It is said that yoga in ancient India was just influenced by this and thereby emerged.

【发展】

公元8世纪,日本从中国引进了足部按摩——"足心道",后者一直为日本民间和医学界所推广运用,日本是一个足部按摩法颇有成就的国家,日本东京工业大学的平泽弥一郎教授有"脚底博士"的绰号,他对脚的研究大约有40多年,至少接触过2万人的脚。20世纪的美国的鲍尔博士将菲特兹格拉得的区带疗法总结、撰写成《区带治疗法》,此书对后来足疗的发展起了重要的作用。20世纪50年代德国的一位女士受《脚会说话》一书的影响,经过学习、研究、总结出版《足反射疗法》,此书流传到东西方的国家,它使足部按摩疗法风靡世界,足部反射区疗法也已基本成形。

【回归】

吴若石神父是我国台湾省瑞士籍的传教士,曾患膝关节炎,在中西医治疗无效的情况下,自学《足部反射区病理按摩法》一书,后自治膝关节炎3次,膝关节就好了,于是他对这种按摩法产生浓厚的兴趣,开始学习研究之,并请人把此书由德文译成中文,取名《病理按摩法》。此按摩法首先在台湾引起震动,为此他在台湾省成立了"若石健康研究会",把该按摩法中的50多个反射区,发展为62个,除作理论研究外,还对足反射区按摩进行大力推广和宣传。

随着我国的改革开放,吴若石的学生将足部反射区按摩法带至北京,并向全国推广。足部反射区按摩法也就重新回到了祖国大

Development

In 8th century A.D., Japanese people introduced foot massage from China and formed "Sokushindo", which has been applied and popularized among Japanese folks and medical experts. Japan is a country with great achievements of foot massage. Take for example Yayichirou Hirasawa at Tokyo Institute of Technology in Japan. He has got a nickname "Dr. Sole of Foot", for he has about 40 years' experiences in research on foot and has touched at least 20, 000 person's feet. In early 20th century, Dr. Edwin Bowers in the United States summarized William Fitzgerald's theory of zone therapy and composed *Zone Therapy*, which played a significant role in the further development of foot therapy. In 1950s, a woman in Germany, who was influenced by a book entitled *Foot Speaks*, started to study, examine, and summarize foot massage, and finally published *Foot Reflexology*. This book was later spread to western and eastern countries and gradually made foot massage popular throughout the world. Accordingly, foot reflex zone massage came into being on the whole.

Regression

Father Wu Rwo-Shur (originally named Father Josef Eugster), a Swiss missionary in Taiwan Province, suffered from arthritis in his knees. When western and Chinese medicines were of no efficacy, he began to teach himself a book called *Pathological Massage Method for Foot Reflex Zones*. Later he treated arthritis in his knees by himself for three times, and cured his problems. Then he became strongly interested in foot massage and started to study and examine it. He even had the book translated from German into Chinese, naming it *Pathological Massage Method*. The method first caused a sensation throughout Taiwan. Therefore, he established "Rwo-Shur Health Institute", and went on to develop more than 50 zones in the original massage method into 62 zones. Apart from doing theoretical

陆，现在越来越多医务工作者及非医务工作者对此疗法重视起来，1991年7月经国家卫生部及民政局批准，中国足部反射区疗法健康法研究会正式成立，经卫生部门的认可，定名为"反射疗法"。2002年初，经过卫生部的培训、考核，第一批反射疗法师已经获得认证。

第二节 足部反射区按摩的概念、作用以及与其他疗法的关系

古今中外防病、治病的方法很多，无论是中国的传统医学，西方的现代医学，还是具双重特点的中西医药结合的医学，各自都有其不同的特点，都有其长处。在应用中要取长补短，才能发挥各自特长。

【足部反射区按摩的概念和作用】

足部反射区按摩就是在人体的某一部分，病变部位或器官相对应的反射区，找出敏感点——酸、麻、胀、痛点，加以按摩，

research on foot reflex zone massage, he vigorously publicized the method.

Under the circumstances of reform and opening-up of China, students of Wu Rwo-Shur introduced methods of foot reflex zone massage to Beijing and popularized them throughout the country. Hence, the method of foot reflex zone massage returned to mainland China. Nowadays more and more medical workers and non-medical workers begin to attach importance to the therapy. In July 1991, after being ratified by the Ministry of Health and Civil Administration Bureau, China Institute of Foot Reflex Zone Therapy and Health Method was formally established. And the method was called "Reflex Therapy". In early 2002, having undergone training and examination given by the Ministry of Health, the first group of reflex therapists were certified.

Section 2　Foot Reflex Zone Massage: Conception, Functions, and its Relations with Other Therapies

In modern or ancient times, in China or the rest of the world, there have been plenty of methods to prevent or cure diseases. Different methods have different characteristics and advantages no matter whether they belong to traditional Chinese medicine, modern Western medicine or integrated traditional and Western medicine that combines both features. Only by drawing on each other's merits, can we bring these methods into full play respectively.

Conception and Functions of Foot Reflex Zone Massage

Foot Reflex Zone Massage refers to a therapeutic method that attempts to find and massage tenderness points, i.e. sore, numb, distension, and aching points in the reflex zone on certain region of human body that corresponds to the region or organ with

达到防病治病效果的一种治疗方法。是一种科学性和实用性很强的保健按摩法。不但是男女老少保健的理想方法,而且能治疗许多病痛,甚至能解决别的医疗方法不能见效或不易见效的疾病。此外,在某些病没有显现出来以前,在脚部的某个部位就可有所变化,故此,足部反射区按摩也可作为一种独特的诊疗手段。

足部反射区按摩具有止痛、解除疲劳、诊断疾病、增智及防病保健等作用。

足部反射区按摩的特点是没有药物的副作用、简便,易学,经济。它通过调节神经反射,改善血液循环,调节内分泌,增强免疫系统功能,通经活络等原理,达到扶正祛邪、防病治病的目的。但它仅仅是医疗保健的一种方法,有一定的局限性,它不是能取代其他疗法的灵丹妙药。我们要发挥其特长,不排斥其他的治疗方法。

【足部反射区按摩与其他疗法的关系】

首先它可以减少因服药和手术造成的副作用。因为经常做足部反射区按摩可以增强机体的免疫和抵抗力。其次它对术后患者

pathological changes, so as to produce efficacy of preventing or curing diseases. It is a scientific and practical massage method for health preservation. It is not only the ideal method for men and women, the young and the old, to keep health, but also the one capable of curing many diseases, even those disorders on which other medical methods can hardly or not produce curative effects. In addition, prior to manifestations of some conditions, there are already some changes on certain region of the feet. Therefore, foot reflex zone massage can be used as a unique diagnostic and therapeutic means.

Foot Reflex Zone Massage can stop pain, relieve fatigue, diagnose disease, enhance intelligence, prevent illness and preserve health.

Foot Reflex Zone Massage is characterized by absence of side-effect of medications, simple, minimal cost, and easy to learn. Through the principle of regulating nervous reflex, improving blood circulation, adjusting endocrine secretion, enhancing functions of immunologic system, and activating meridians and collaterals, etc., it helps to strengthen healthy qi to eliminate pathogens, and prevent and cure diseases. However, it is only one of the methods of medical treatment and health care, with certain limitations. It is not the panacea capable of replacing other therapies. We need to bring its virtues into full play, without rejecting other therapeutic methods.

The Relation between Foot Reflex Zone Massage and Other Therapies

First of all, it can diminish the side effect of drugs or operations, since frequently massaging foot reflex zones can enhance the body's immunity and resistance. Secondly, for the patient after operation, it helps to make the affected region recover quickly, hence speeding up the rehabilitation of the patient. And for the

可使病变部位早日恢复，可以缩短患者的康复时间。对于有急性感染患者，经常在敏感区做足部反射区按摩再配合药物治疗，也可使用药疗程缩短，同时可减少药物的副作用，减轻患者的痛苦，缩短康复时间。总之它和其他治疗方法并不矛盾，可相互补充，相互协助，以发挥各自独特的治疗保健作用。

第三节 足部反射区按摩的入门要领

【怎样入门】

第一、掌握足部反射区的分布规律：足部反射区有一定的规律性，两只脚并起来是一个坐着的人。

第二、按系统记忆反射区：如肾脏、输尿管、膀胱、尿道是泌尿系统；胃、十二指肠、小肠、结肠、肛门是消化系统。

第三、分次记：每次记几个反射区，背熟后再记几个反射区，日积月累，积少成多。

第四、边学边练。这是最好的一种学习方法，最好两人一起做。

第五、带着问题学习更能提高效率。

足部反射区按摩是一个由生到熟、由慢到快的过程，这个过程

patient with acute infection, constantly massaging the foot reflex zones in the tenderness areas by combining drugs can also reduce the course of treatment. At the same time, it can diminish the side effect of drugs, alleviate the pains of the patients, speed up rehabilitation. In a word, it does not contradict other therapies. And they can complement and coordinate with each other, so as to bring their own special functions of treatment and health care into full play.

Section 3 The Rudimentary Essentials of Foot Reflex Zone Massage

Beginner's Guide

First, Grasp the distribution law of reflex zones: There is certain rules of foot reflex zones. For instance, two feet closed together shape like a sitting person.

Secondly, Memorize the reflex zones according to the systems. For example, kidney, ureter, bladder and urethra belong to urinary system; stomach, duodenum, small intestine, colon and anus belong to digestive system.

Thirdly, Memorize at different times: memorize several reflex zones each time. After learning them by heart, go on to memorize other reflex zones. You will remember more and more reflex zones with the accumulation over a long period of time.

Fourthly, Practice while learning. This the best learning method, most suitable for two persons to work together.

Fifthly, Learning by bearing question in mind is easier to improve efficiency.

Foot reflex zone massage is a process that ranges from unskilled to skillful, from slow to fast. It is also an accumulated, progressive one and therefore you need to be patient. In order to achieve good efficacy, you must undergone long period of exploration and master

是一个积累、循序渐进的过程,不能性急,要有耐心,要按客观规律办事。要取得好的治疗效果,必须经过长时间的摸索,掌握足部反射区按摩手法在一定反射区的特点,才会有收获。不能怕苦怕累、怕没有效果,要持之以恒。

【按摩的顺序、方向、时间】

1. 按摩顺序:原则上应先左后右;先足底,再足内侧、足外侧、足背。多从心脏反射区开始,然后做排泄系统。此外,还要按由远至近的顺序。

2. 按摩方向:主张由远至近的按摩方向,因为这样既有利于血液及淋巴的回流,排除毒素,又有利于记忆。

3. 按摩时间:每个按摩区平均按摩10~30秒。力量由轻到重,逐渐增加,每只脚最少按10多分钟,最多25分钟。

【注意事项】

1. 按摩的场合要空气新鲜、温度适中。

2. 术者操作前要洗手,剪手指甲。

3. 接受按摩者在洗脚时剪短脚趾甲、修磨过厚的脚垫。有足癣先抹药膏再按摩。

4. 按摩前先观察对方的健康状态,了解两点:①保健重点。②耐受情况。

the features of the manipulations of foot reflex zone massage in a given reflex zone. Only by doing so can you learn something. Perseverence is essential to learn this therapy.

The Order, Direction and Time of Massage

1. Order of Massage: In principle, You should start from left to right; from the sole of the foot through the interior aspect of the foot and exterior aspect of the foot to the back of foot. People usually start from heart reflex zone, then to the excretory system. In addition, you should pay attention to the order from distal to local areas.

2. Direction of Massage: It is recommended to massage in the direction from distal to local areas, which is beneficial to memory as well as reflux of blood and lymph, and expelling of toxin.

3. Time of Massage: Massage averagely 10-30 seconds in each massage zone, with gradually increasing force. You better massage each foot 10-25 minutes.

Precautions

1. The place where massage is done requires fresh air and moderate temperature.

2. The doctor should wash his or her hands, and trim his or her fingernails before operating.

3. The person who receives massage should trim short his or her toenails and rub his or her foot callus. Those who have ringworm of feet should administer ointment before taking massage.

4. The masseur should first observe the health state of the patient in order to make sure two points: ① the important points of health care. ② the degree of tolerance.

5. During massage, you should understand the reaction or demand of the patient at any time, and frequently adjust the stimulation.

6. Be prudent for those who are in relatively severe state of

5. 按摩中要随时了解对方的反应和要求，经常调整刺激量。

6. 对病情较重或没有把握估计预后者应慎重从事。既不要无根据地下判断，也不要马上停止原来的用药和治疗。

7. 对足踝外伤肿胀不能用热水泡脚，应先冷敷，止痛，待24小时后再进行按摩。

8. 对出血性疾病应谨慎从事，或采用轻手法或不予按摩。

9. 早孕或危重患者慎施按摩。

10. 对诊断不清或癌症患者，按摩者一定要向患者解释清楚相关事项，患者坚持按摩时，按摩者要与患者或家属分清责任。

11. 按摩前后患者要饮水300～500毫升，有利于排出毒素。

12. 按摩后征求患者意见和反映，并用消毒水洗手，以防止感染。

总之，在做足部反射区按摩时注意以上事项能提高治疗效果，避免不良后果。

illness or those with unknown prognosis. Neither make judgment without grounds nor suspend original medications or treatment.

7. For those who suffer from external injury or swelling of ankles, you must not immerse their feet in hot water. You should first apply cold compress so as to stop pain, and then massage after 24 hours.

8. For those who suffer from hemorrhagic diseases, be cautious when massaging. Or adopt light manipulations or not to massage.

9. For the patients who are in early pregnancy or critical conditions, generally not massage.

10. For the patient without clear diagnosis or with cancer, the masseur is required to explain benefits and potential risks clearly to the patients. If the patient insists on being massaged, the masseur and the patient's family members should make sure who should be responsible for the results.

11. Before massage, the patient should drink 300-500 milliliter of water, which is beneficial to expel toxins.

12. After massage, you should communicate with the patient and wash your hands with antiseptic solution for fear of mycotic infection.

In a word, you are able to improve therapeutic efficacy and avoid bad consequences by paying attention to the above-mentioned precautions when doing foot reflex zone massage.

第二章 | 足部反射区按摩的医学原理

足部反射区按摩,它的神奇功效是有目共睹的。为什么会有这样的作用呢?医学家们在实践中,结合现代科学理论知识,经研究和分析后发现,足部反射区按摩和以下理论联系密切。

第一节 阴阳平衡理论

世界万物是一个阴阳的平衡体,它的生长和变化都遵循阴阳平衡的规律,人体内的一切生命活动也离不开瞬息万变的阴阳变化,生为阳,死为阴;动为阳,静为阴;阴阳的不断变化促进了生命的生长,因为有人体内阴阳的不同变化,也就造成了人体外发生不同的变化——生病。足部反射区按摩就是通过按摩刺激不同反射区来调节人体内阴阳,起到平衡阴阳的作用,达到防病治病的目的。以失眠为例,导致此病的原因多是由于大脑过度紧张造成的,属于阳盛,以轻柔缓和的手法按摩足部的脑反射区和其他相关反射区,可以使大脑得到放松,改变它的紧张状态,即给大脑一个阴柔的信号来代替阳刚的信息,达到平衡阴阳的作用。

Chapter 2 The Medical Principles of Foot Reflex Zone Massage

The marvelous effectiveness of foot reflex zone massage is well-known. Why does it have such efficacy? In the course of practice, medical experts made research and analyses by integrating with modern theory and scientific knowledge, and discovered that foot reflex zone massage is closely related to the following theories.

Section 1 The Theory of Balance between Yin and Yang

All things in the world are an entity of yin-yang balance. All the life activities within human body cannot perform without myriad changes of yin and yang. For instance, life is yang and death is yin; motion is yang and stillness is yin. The constant changing of yin and yang promote the growth of life. Since there are different changes of yin and yang within human body, there are accordingly different changes that occur in the interior and exterior of human body, i.e. diseases. Foot reflex zone massage is used to regulate yin and yang by massaging and stimulating different reflex zones, so as to perform the function of balancing yin and yang, and achieve the goal of preventing and curing diseases. Take insomnia for example, the disorder is mainly caused by overstrain of the brain, which belongs to yang. Therefore, massaging the brain reflex zone on the foot and other related reflex zones with light, soft and gentle manipulations can relax the brain and change the mental stress, i.e. sending a yin and soft signal to the brain in place of the information of yang and rigid, so as to balance yin and yang.

第二节 神经反射学说

人体是一个复杂的，但各部位、各器官又互相联系的有机整体。各部位或各器官有规律的分布在足部周围。在按摩足部某一反射区时，通过神经反射作用与某一相对应部位或器官发生联系，也就是说一种刺激通过足部的反射区神经到达了相应的病变区或需要调节的脏腑，起到了防病治病的作用。相反，如果某一器官有病也会在一定的反射区有所表现，如心肌缺氧时，足部的心脏反射区会出现反应点或疼痛；子宫切除后在子宫的反射区会出现空虚感；乳腺肿瘤在其反射区可摸到结节等。

第三节 血液循环原理

人体的血液循环担负着为全身各器官组织输送养分、氧气和将代谢产物及二氧化碳排出体外的任务。足部处于全身最低的位置，离心脏最远，血液的流速最慢，再加上地心的引力，血液中的酸性代谢产物和未被利用的矿物质钙等容易沉积下来，日积月累，足部就成了最需要清除沉积物的部位。沉积物过多地积存于某一个反射区时，该反射区就会产生反应，发生一定的变化，如结节、空虚、疼痛等等。足部反射区按摩可以改善足部的血循环及促进器官组织的新陈代谢，增强组织细胞的活动，可以说足部反射区按摩在血液循环中起了"泵血"的作用，有人称之为"第二心脏"。

Section 2 The Doctrine of Nervous Reflex

Human body is a complex organic whole with interacted areas and organs. Different parts and organs are regularly distributed around the feet. When massaging a certain foot reflex zone, it will be connected to a corresponding part or organ through nervous reflex. That is to say, one stimulus reaches the corresponding affected region or viscerum that needs to be regulated, so as to prevent and cure disorders. On the contrary, if one organ is affected, it will be manifested in a given reflex zone. For example, when the cardiac muscle is lacking oxygen, the reaction point will appear and ache will be felt in the heart reflex zone on the foot; after hysterectomia, the uterus reflex zone give a feeling of voidness; for breast tumor, nodule can be touched in the breast reflex zone.

Section 3 The Principle of Blood Circulation

Blood circulation in human body is responsible for transporting nutrient and oxygen to every organ and tissue in the whole body and discharge products of metabolism and carbon dioxide out of the body. The feet are located at the lowest position of the body and are the farthest from the heart, which leads to the slowest flow of blood. In addition, there exists terrestrial gravity. Besides, the acid products of metabolism and the mineral calcium in the blood are easily to deposit. All these things, after accumulating for a long period of time, give rise to the fact that the feet become the foremost parts from which deposit needs to be eliminated. When too much deposit accumulates in a certain reflex zone, the reflex zone will respond accordingly, with occurrence of certain changes such as nodule, voidness and pain, etc. Foot reflex zone massage can improve blood circulation of feet, promote the metabolism of organs and tissues, and enhance the activities of histological cells. In a certain sense,

第四节 经络学说

经络学说是中医学基础理论之一，它是客观存在的但又不能为肉眼所看到。经络学说认为经络就是起到连接上下肢体，沟通脏腑内外的通道，足部有38个穴位，与足部的反射区基本一致，如涌泉穴为肾经的起点穴位，位置与反射区的肾与肾上腺反射区一致；侠溪穴治偏头痛、耳鸣，在足部反射区中正好位于平衡器官反射区；太溪、照海和子宫、尿道反射区位置相近，功能也类似。足部反射区按摩也讲"得气"，与针灸刺法中的"得气"有着相同的感觉，虽然方法不同，但效果是一样的。因此，足部反射按摩也是通过经络这个通道发挥作用，达到疏经通络，调节脏腑，平衡阴阳的目的。

foot reflex zone massage functions "pumping blood" in blood circulation. Hence, it is called "the second heart".

Section 4 The Theory of Meridians and Collaterals

The theory of meridians and collaterals is one of the basic theories of traditional Chinese medicine. Meridians and collaterals exist objectively but cannot be seen by naked eyes. They are pathways that link the upper limbs with the lower limbs, the upper part of the body with the lower part of the body, and connect the interior with exterior of viscera. There are 38 acupoints on foot, which are generally consistent with foot reflex zones. For instance, Yongquan(KI 1) is the starting point of kidney meridian. Its position is consistent with reflex zones that correspond to kidney and adrenal gland; Xiaxi(GB 43) is to treat migraine and tinnitus. In foot reflex zones, it happens to be situated in the reflex zone corresponding to balancing organ. Taixi(KI 3) and Zhaohai(KI 6) are nearly located in the reflex zones to uterus and urethra respectively, and have similar functions to them. Foot reflex massage also talks about "arrival of qi", which is the same as the "arrival of qi" in acupuncture. Although the methods are different, the effects are the same. Therefore, foot reflex massage also performs functions through the pathways, meridians and collaterals, so as to dredge meridians and collaterals, regulate viscera, and balance yin and yang.

第五节 生物全息论学说

在自然界中每一个局部都包含它自身在内的整体的全部信息。如地球有太阳系的全部信息，太阳系有整个宇宙的全部信息。生物体也一样，人体的每一个局部都有整体的信息。正如一个受精卵，它的细胞核内包含了父母所赋予的全部生物信息，在发育中细胞一分为二，二分四……每个细胞都包含有与受精卵细胞相同的生物信息，最后发育成一个复杂的有许多器官组成的有机体后，每个局部也仍然包含着整个机体的全部信息。耳、鼻、手、脚和头都是这样的局部，它们都是全身的缩影，针灸学的"耳针"、"头针"、"鼻针"都是以此为理论基础的，足部反射区按摩亦然。

第六节 心理作用

医学模式的转变使人们更重视心理因素对人体的影响。人随时可能受到来自外界环境的干扰，同时也受喜、怒、忧、思、悲、恐、惊等七情的制约。中医有"怒伤肝，喜伤心，思伤脾，忧伤肺，恐伤肾"之说。现代社会，人们需要在竞争中求生存，在这错综复杂的社会环境中，每个人都承担不同程度的心理压力。如果这种压力长期得不到缓解，可能影响到人体的脏腑功能及免疫系统，从而进一步造成疾病的产生。由于精神紧张造成的失眠、消化不良、高血压、心脏病等为数不少。足部反射区按摩可使被按摩者得到良好的心理治疗：首先，足部反射区按摩通过促进了下肢的血液循环并减轻了头部的压力，可缓解大脑神经的

Section 5 The Doctrine of Biological Hologram

In the natural world, each part contains all the information of the whole including itself. For instance, the earth contains all the information of the solar system, and the solar system all the information of the whole universe. So is the living body. Each part of the human body contains all the information of the whole, just like a fertilized egg, the cellular nucleus of which contains all the bioinformation granted the parents. In the process of growth, the cell splits in two, and two split in four...Each cell contains the same bioinformation as that of the fertilized egg cell. The process goes on until developing into a complex organism which is composed of many organs. But each part still contains all the information of the whole organism. The ear, nose, hands, feet and head all belongs to such parts. All of them are the miniature of the whole body. All of "ear needle", "scalp needle", and "nose needle" in the study of acupuncture and moxibustion are based on the theory, so is foot reflex zone massage.

Section 6 Psychological Effect

The change of the medical model makes people attach more importance to the influence of psychological factors on human body. Humans are often interfered by the external environment and the seven emotions, i.e. joy, anger, anxiety, pensiveness, grief, fear and fright. Traditional Chinese medicine asserts that "Anger impairs the liver, joy the heart, pensiveness the spleen, anxiety the lung, and fear the kidney". In modern society, people need to survive in competition. In such complicated social environment, each person is burdened with psychological stress at different levels. If such stress is not relieved for a long period of time, it may impact on the functions

紧张状况；其次，足部反射区按摩通过加速大脑氧气的转换过程，具有一定的提神作用；再次，足部反射区按摩又是一种精神抚慰剂，它可使按摩者从精神上得到一定安慰，使其增加一种健康向上的动力，从而增强其克服工作困难或疾病的信心。如果是自己的亲人或朋友为自己做按摩，这种心理作用会更强烈。

of viscera and the immune system, which in turn leads to diseases. There are many cases of insomnia, indigestion, hypertension and heart disease, etc. that are caused by mental stress. Foot reflex zone massage is capable of giving the massaged good psychotherapy. First of all, foot reflex zone massage lessens the stress of the head by promoting the blood circulation of the lower limbs, which helps relieve the tense condition of cerebral nerves. Secondly, foot reflex zone massage performs a certain function of refreshment. Thirdly, foot reflex zone massage is a kind of mental soothing agent, which makes the massaged somewhat comforted mentally and gain a certain kind of motive power that is healthy and positive, thereby strengthening his or her confidence in overcoming working difficulties or diseases. If it is his or her relative or friend that is massaging the massaged, the psychological effect will be stronger.

第三章 足部反射区定位和操作

第一节 足部反射区大体定位与对应关系以及按摩手法

【足部反射区定位概述】

我们已经知道，人体的各脏腑器官，在足部都有其相对应的反射区。这些反射区是如何定位的呢？根据我们看到的资料，各国学者曾提出过许多不同的反射图。由于篇幅关系，我们只介绍其中几种，目的是说明一个问题，反射区的定位并不是那么绝对的、唯一的。不同的学派可能有不同的划分法。这种认识上的差异并不奇怪，因为认识上的差异反映了实际情况上的差异。人与人之间本来就存在着差异，脚与脚不可能一模一样，尺寸大小形状比例各不相同，并不是一种几何相似图形的放大或缩小。而且，人们对体表敏感点的发现和认识也有一个发展的过程，这个过程至今还没有终结。因此，我们在对反射区进行定位时，应考虑到实际情况的复杂性，不能像划国界省界那样去划分反射区的边界，或者采取几何投影的办法去精确地确定反射区的坐标，而宜于采取某种"模糊逻辑"的方法，以我们对脏腑器官与体表敏感点相互对应关系的感性经验为基础，对每个反射区大体上规定一个范围，指出各个反射区的相对位置。搞清每个反射区的相对位置，这是进行按摩诊治和自我保健的前提条件，是掌握足部反射区健康法的首要基本功，每位学员都应牢牢记住（《用足部反

Chapter 3 Location and Operation of Foot Reflex Zones

Section 1 Foot Reflex Zones: Rough Location, Corresponding relations and Manipulations of Massage

A General Overview of Positioning of Foot Reflex Zones

We have already known that every viscerum in human body has its corresponding reflex zone on the feet. Then how to locate these reflex zones? According to the data we have collected, scholars from different countries put forward different charts of reflex zones. Due to the limited space, we only introduce a few of them. The purpose is to elucidate a problem that the location of reflex zones is not necessarily abstract and exclusive, and different schools may have different dividing methods. It is not strange to have such disparities in cognition, which reflect the differences in actual situation. There always exist differences between people. For example, it is impossible for human feet to look exactly alike. And these feet may have different size, shape and proportion, and they are not simply the magnification or minification of a certain geometric figure. Moreover, there is a course of development for people to discover and get to know the tenderness points on the surface of the human body. This course is not over yet. Therefore, when we position the reflex zones, we should take into account the complexity of the actual situation. We should neither divide the borders of the reflex zones like dividing national or

射疗法帮助你自己》1969年美国Mildred Carter)。

尽管有60多个反射区,要记住这些反射区的相对位置并不是很困难的事,因为这些反射区的位置并不是胡乱确定,毫无规律可循的。它是人们长期实践观察的总结,有一定的规律性。我们可用下面的示意图来说明足部反射区的定位,帮助我们掌握每个反射区的相对位置。

如图1、图2所示,双脚并拢在一起,可以看成是一个坐着的人形。脚的踇趾,相当于人的头部。脚底的前半部,相当于人的胸部(有肺及心脏)。脚的外侧,自上而下是肩、肘、膝等部位。脚底的中部,相当于人的腹部,有胃、肠、胰、肝胆(右侧)、脾(左侧)、肾等器官。脚跟部分,相当于盆腔,有生殖器官(子宫、卵巢、前列腺)、膀胱、尿道(阴道)、肛门等。脚的内侧,构成足弓的一条线,相当于人的脊椎(颈椎-胸椎-腰椎-骶骨)。

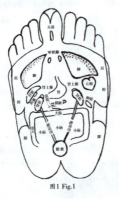

图1 Fig.1

甲状腺: thyroid gland 肩: shoulder 肺: lung 肘: elbow 肝胆: liver 肾上腺: adrenal gland 心脏: heart 胆囊: gall 肾脏: kidney 胃: stomach 胰脏: pancreas 脾脏: spleen 十二指肠: duodenum 大肠: large intestine 小肠: small intestine 输尿管: ureter 膀胱: bladder

provincial boundaries, nor precisely determine the coordinate of the reflex zone by means of geometric projection. Instead, we should take the method of "fuzzy logic", roughly diving a sphere for each reflex zone and pointing out the relative position of each reflex zone, on the basis of the sensible experience we have got about the mutual corresponding relations between viscera and the tenderness points on the body surface. Making clear the relative location of each reflex zone is not only the prerequisite of performing massage diagnosis and therapy and self health care, but also the first and foremost basic skill to master foot reflex zone healthy method. Every student should keep it firmly in mind (*Helping Yourself with Foot Reflexology* by Mildred Carter in the U.S. in 1969).

Although there are more than 60 reflex zones. It is not very difficult to memorize the relative positions of these reflex zones, because the locations of these reflex zones are distributed on rules. It has been summarized through long term of practice and observation. We can explain the location of foot reflex zones with the following sketch so as to help us master the relative location of each reflex zone.

As is shown in Fig. 1 and Fig. 2, put the two feet close side by side, which can be regarded as a sitting human figure. The big toe amounts to the human head, the front part of the soles of the feet amounts to the human chest (with the lungs and heart). Along the medial aspects of the feet, there are zones that correspond to the places such as the shoulders, elbows and knees from above to below. The middle part of the soles amounts to the abdomen, in which there are the organs such as stomach, intestines, liver and gall (right), spleen (left), kidney. The heels amount to cavity of pelvis, in which there are reproductive organs (uterus, ovaries, prostate glands), bladders,

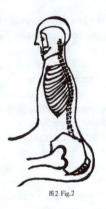

图2 Fig.2

以上漫画式的描述,只是为了使大家有一个总的概念。以下我们将大致上按照按摩的顺序,逐一介绍每一个反射区,使学习者有较详尽的了解。在文中所用的方位术语,将按照解剖学的一般规定:对人体来说,头部的方向为上,脚的方向为下;腹部的一侧为前,背部的一侧为后;以身体正中面为基准,距正中面近者为内侧,距正中面远者为外侧。上肢以拇指一侧为外侧(桡侧),小指一侧为内侧(尺侧)。下肢以踇趾一侧为内侧(胫侧)、小趾一侧为外侧(腓侧)。 对脚部来说,脚背的一面为上,脚底的一面为下;脚趾的方向为前,脚跟的方向为后;踇趾一侧为内,小趾一侧为外。图3、图4所示为足部反射区的示意图。

urethra (vagina), anus. The medial aspect of the feet makes up a line of instep, which amounts to human's vertebra (cervical vertebra, thoracic vertebra, lumbar vertebra, terminal vertebra).

The above cartoon-like description is only used to make you have a general overview. Then we will start to introduce each reflex zone roughly in accordance with the order of massage, making learners have a thorough knowledge of reflex zones. The terms for locations used in the text conform to the regulations of anatomy: for human body, the direction of the head is superior, while the direction of the feet is inferior; abdomen aspect is anterior, while the back aspect is posterior; benchmarked by the middlemost surface of the body, what is close to the middlemost surface is called medial surface, while what is far from the middlemost surface is called lateral surface. For the upper limbs, the thumb aspect is regarded as lateral surface (radial surface), while the little finger aspect is called the medial surface (ulnar surface). For the lower limbs, the big toe aspect is called medial surface (tibial surface), while the little toe aspect is called the lateral surface (fibula surface). For the foot, the dorsum aspect is called superior, while the sole aspect is called inferior; the direction of the toes is called anterior, while the direction of the heel is called posterior; the big toe aspect is called medial, while the little toe aspect is called lateral. Fig. 3 and Fig. 4 show the sketch diagram of foot reflex zones.

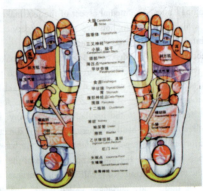

图3 Fig.3

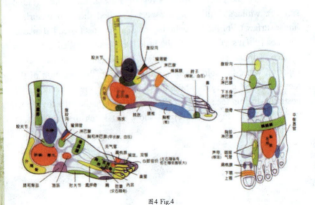

图4 Fig.4

(左脚内侧) (The medial surface of the left foot)

直肠：rectum 髋关节：hip joint 腹股沟：groin 输卵管：fallopian tube 淋巴管：lymphoduct 横膈膜：diaphragm 脑干：brain stem 鼻：nose 内尾骨：internal coccyx 膀胱：bladder 颈椎：cervical vertebra 胸椎：thoracic vertebra 腰椎：lumbar vertebra 骶椎：sacral vertebra 痔疾：hemorrhoids

(右脚外侧) (The lateral surface of the right foot)

髋关节：hip joint 腹股沟：groin 输卵管：oviduct 淋巴管：lymphoduct 胸部淋巴腺：thoracic lymph gland （甲状腺：thyroid gland 血压：blood pressure) 直肠：rectum 肘关节：elbow joint 肩胛骨：scapula 内耳：inner ear 支气管：bronchus 盲肠：cecum 横膈膜：diaphragm 内尾骨：internal coccyx 扁桃腺：tonsil

（左脚背）(The dorsum of left foot)

腹股沟：groin 肋骨 ribs 上半身淋巴腺：lymph gland in the upper body 下半身淋巴腺：lymph gland in the lower body 胸部淋巴腺：thoracic lymph gland 上颚：upper jaw 下颚：lower jaw 声带：vocal cord 咽喉：throat 气管：trachea 扁桃腺：tonsil 平衡器官：balancing organ 横膈膜：diaphragm

【足部反射区按摩手法】

(一) 常用手法

足部反射区按摩的手法有10多种,最常用的是示指(食指)扣拳法和拇指推法,现介绍如下:

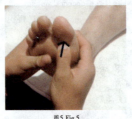

图5 Fig.5

拇指按压法(图5):

1. 着力点:拇指指腹。

2. 施力部位:手腕、手掌。

3. 适用反射区:内肋骨、外肋骨、喉、解溪、气管和腹股沟等。

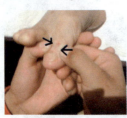

图6 Fig.6

拇指扣指法(图6):

1. 着力点:拇指指尖处。指尖与皮肤垂直。

2. 施力部位:拇指指间关节、手掌、腕关节。

3. 适用反射区:三叉神经、鼻、颈椎、扁桃腺、上颚、副甲状腺。

拇指推法(图7):

1. 着力点:拇指指腹。

2. 施力部位:手掌、腕关节。

3. 适用反射区:尿道、三叉神经、颈项、胸椎、腰椎、骶椎、内侧坐骨神经、横膈膜、食管和气管等。

Manipulations of Foot Reflex Massage

Ⅰ. Commonly used Manipulations

There are more than 10 manipulations of foot reflex massage. The most common ones are buckling fist with the index finger, and pushing with the thumb.

Pressing manipulation with the thumb(Fig.5):
1. Point of exerting force: finger pulp of the thumb.
2. Place of exerting force: the wrist and palm.
3. Indicated reflex zones: internal or external ribs, larynx, Jiexi (ST 41), windpipe, groin, etc.

Buckling manipulation with the thumb(Fig.6):
1. Point of exerting force: the tip of the thumb, which is perpendicular to the skin.
2. Place of exerting force: interphalangeal joint of the thumb, palm, and wrist joint.
3. Indicated reflex zones: trigeminal nerve, nose, cervical vertebra, tonsil, palate, accessory thyroid gland.

Pushing manipulation with the thumb(Fig. 7):
1. Point of exerting force: finger pulp of the thumb.
2. Place of exerting force: palm and wrist joint.
3. Indicated reflex zones: urinary canal, trigeminal nerve, neck, thoracic, lumbar or sacral vertebra, medial sciatic nerve, diaphragm, esophagus and trachea.

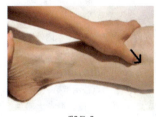

图7 Fig.7

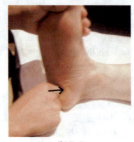
图8 Fig.8

示指扣拳法（图8）：

1. 着力点：示指第二指骨间关节背面尺侧突起部。

2. 施力部位：手腕、拳背。

3. 适用反射区：肾上腺、肾、小脑和脑干、大脑、副甲状腺、额窦、斜方肌、心、脾、胃、胰、小肠、大肠、肛门、生殖腺、胸椎、腰椎、骶椎、内外侧坐骨神经、肩关节、肘关节、膝关节、下腹部、食管和气管等。

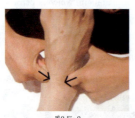
图9 Fig.9

示指钩拳法（图9）：

1. 着力点：示指外侧（桡侧或称虎口侧）。

2. 施力部位：拇指固定，其余三指辅助手掌用力。

3. 适用反射区：甲状腺、前列腺、子宫、髋关节、内外尾骨、生殖腺（卵巢、睾丸等）。

握足扣指法（图10）：

1. 着力点：示指第一指点节背侧。

2. 施力部位：握拳之手腕、另一手拇指为辅助，四指为握足之固点。

Buckling fist manipulation with the index finger (Fig. 8):

1. Point of exerting force: ulnar protrusive part on the dorsal surface of the second interphalangeal joint of the index finger.

2. Place of exerting force: wrist, dorsum of the fist.

3. Indicated reflex zones: adrenal gland, kidney, cerebellum and brain stem, cerebrum, accessory thyroid gland, frontal sinus, trapezius muscle, heart, spleen, stomach, pancreas, small intestine, large intestine, anus, genital gland, thoracic, lumbar, sacral vertebra, medial and lateral sciatic nerves, shoulder joint, elbow joint, knee joint, lower abdomen, esophagus and windpipe.

Hooking fist manipulation with the index finger (Fig. 9):

1. Point of exerting force: lateral aspect of the index finger (also called radial surface or hukou surface).

2. Place of exerting force: fix the thumb with the rest three fingers assisting the palm in exerting force.

3. Indicated reflex zones: thyroid gland, prostate gland, uterus, hip joint, internal and external coccyxes, genital gland (ovary, testicle, etc).

Gripping foot and buckling finger manipulation (Fig. 10):

1. Point of exerting force: dorsal surface of the first knuckle of the index finger.

2. Place of exerting force: wrist of the gripping fist, with the other hand in which the thumb serves as auxiliary, and the four fingers serve as the fix point for gripping the foot.

3. Indicated reflex zones: the key reflex zones or tenderness points to adrenal gland, kidney, etc. that need exertion of force.

3. 适用反射区：肾上腺、肾等需要加力的重点反射区或敏感点。

拳推法 （图11）：

1. 着力点：第二至第五指近侧指骨间关节稍远端。

2. 施力部位：以上臂的力量使拳向前推移。

3. 适用反射区：小腿部外侧的坐骨神经反射区、小肠反射区及通三焦法。

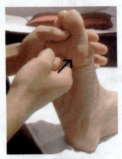

图10 Fig.10

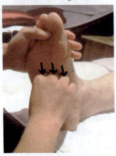

图11 Fig.11

（二）手法的基本要求

足部反射区按摩为了达到调节人体生理功能、防病治病的效果，必须正确和熟练地掌握和运用按摩的手法，也只有按照手法的基本要求做，才能起到事半功倍的效果。

1. 反射区位置要求准确：选准反射区位置是关键，尤其是找准敏感点，是保证疗效的最基本要求。

2. 力度适当：不同的反射区，因其部位不同，局部解剖结构就不同，对按压所能按受的施力强度则不尽相同。当按压达到酸胀、稍痛但又以能忍受时为度。用力太小，达不到保健目的；用力太

Pushing manipulation with fist (Fig. 11):

1. Point of exerting force: distal ends of the proximal interphalangeal joints of 2nd-5th fingers.

2. Place of exerting force: Push the fist forward with the force of the upper arm.

3. Indicated reflex zones: reflex zones to sciatic nerve on lateral aspect of the lower leg, small intestine and triple energizer.

II. The Basic Requirement of Manipulations

The foot reflex zone massage is used to achieve the effect of regulating physiological functions of human body, and preventing and curing diseases. One must master and perform massage manipulations correctly and skillfully. Only by performing in accordance with the basic requirement of manipulations can one get twice the result with half the effort.

1. Accurate location of the reflex zones: It is of crucial importance to locate reflex zones correctly, especially finding the tenderness point precisely, which is the basic requirement to secure the curative effect.

2. Proper strength: In view of their different corresponding regions, different reflex zones have different topographical structures. Therefore, they require different strength of force. It is appropriate to press to the point of feeling sore and numb with tolerable pain. Too light force may not achieve the health-care effect, whereas too strong stimulation may damage the skeletons, periosts, tendons, muscles, blood vessels and nerves. Through much practical performance, one can master the moderate force supposed to be exerted at different reflex zones. There is another saying that different intensities of force may have the reinforcing or reducing effect. And reinforcing is achieved by exerting relatively weak force to the extent of feeling sore and distending with slight but comfortable pain reducing is

大，易损伤骨骼、骨膜、肌腱、肌肉、血管、神经等。通过较多的实践操作，便可掌握不同反射区一般应施的中等力度。又有一种以力度分补泻的说法，认为用力略小，感到酸胀，稍痛，但较舒适者为补；用力较大，感到疼痛，几乎接近不能忍耐为泻。

3. 施力均匀：对一个反射区，一般要做3～6次。施力可用由小逐渐增大，亦可以基本保持一致，但在一次推按中，要保持施力均匀。也就是说，每做一次推按，先决定这次推按的力度，并将这一力度保持到这次推按的结束，不要忽轻忽重，头轻尾重或头重尾轻。

4. 要有节奏感：在按摩的反射区寻到一个有规律的刺激，使其感到轻松、愉快，有节奏感地施力与放松，而不易感到疲劳。

5. 姿势要正确：掌握正确姿势，既是为了按摩的方便，也是为了按摩轻松、自如。

6. 全身放松：按摩时要注意全身放松，注意力要集中，心情愉快，对效果充满信心，这样对健康有益，有助于提高疗效。

（三）双足反射区按摩顺序

按摩顺序为：左足足底 >左足内侧 >左足外侧 >左足背 >右足底 >右足内侧 >右足外侧 >右足背。各部分具体按摩顺序分述如下：

左足足底：先检查心脏反射区。然后按照以下顺序进行按摩：

1. 肾上腺→2.腹腔反射区→3.肾脏→4.输尿管→5.膀胱→6.尿道→7.前额→8.三叉神经→9.小脑和脑干→10.颈项→11.鼻→12.大脑→13.脑垂体→14.食管和气管→15.甲状旁腺→16.甲状腺→17.其他趾额窦→18.眼→19.耳→20.斜方肌→23.脾→24.胃→25.胰→26.十二

achieved by exerting relatively strong force to the extent of feeling almost intolerable pain.

3. Even exertion of force: For one reflex zone, massage is generally required to be performed 3–6 times. And force can be exerted gradually from weak to strong, or remain roughly the same. But in each pushing and pressing, the force should be kept evenly. That is to say, for each pushing and pressing, the intensity of the force should be determined at first, and the intensity of the force should be maintained till the end of this pushing and pressing, neither sudden lightness nor sudden heaviness, and neither lightness at first and heaviness in the end, nor heaviness at first and lightness in the end.

4. Rhythmical sense: A regular stimulus should be applied to the reflex zone of massage, making the zone feel relaxed and pleasant. Exertion and release of force should be given rhythmically, so as not to cause fatigue.

5. Correct posture: Master the correct posture in order to massage easily and smoothly.

6. Relaxing all over the body: When massaging, one should attach importance to the relaxation of the whole body, concentration, pleasant state of mind, full confidence in the efficacy. These are beneficial to the both health and treatment effect.

III. Massage Order of the Reflex Zones of the Feet

The massage order is: the sole of the left foot→medial surface of the left foot→lateral surface of the left foot→dorsum of the left foot→ the sole of the right foot→medial surface of the right foot→lateral surface of the right foot→dorsum of the right foot. The detailed massage orders of every zones are stated separately as follows:

The sole of the left foot: First examine the heart reflex zone. Then massage in line with the following order:

1. adrenal gland→2. abdominal cavity reflex zone→3. kidney→

指肠→27.小肠→28.横结肠→29.降结肠→30.乙状结肠和直肠→31.肛门→32.生殖腺→33.失眠点→34.止泻点。

左足内侧:

1.颈椎→2.胸椎→3.腰椎→4.骶椎→5.内尾骨→6.子宫或前列腺→7.内肋骨→8.腹股沟→9.下身淋巴结→10.内侧髋关节→11.内侧直肠和肛门→12.内侧坐骨神经。

左足外侧:

1.肩→2.上臂→3.肘→4.膝→5.外尾骨→6.外生殖腺→7.肩胛骨→8.外肋骨→9.上身淋巴结→10.外侧髋关节→11.下腹部→12.外侧坐骨神经。

左足背:

1.上颚→2.下颚→3.扁桃腺→4.咽喉→5.胸部淋巴腺→6.气管→7.内耳→8.胸部和乳房→9.膈肌→10.输尿管和输精管→11.上、下身淋巴结→12.解溪。

右足

右足底:

1.肾上腺→2.腹腔神经丛→3.肾脏→4.输尿管→5.膀胱→6.尿道(会阴)→7.前额(额窦)→8.三叉神经→9.小脑和脑干→10.颈项→11.鼻→12.大脑→13.脑垂体→14.食管和气管→15.甲状旁腺→16.甲状腺→17.其他趾额窦(头部)→18.眼→19.耳→20.斜方肌→21.肺和支气管→22.肝脏→23.胆囊→24.胃→25.胰→26.十二指肠→27.小肠→28.盲肠和阑尾→29.回盲瓣→30.升结肠→31.横结肠→32.生殖腺→33.失眠点→34.止泻点。

4. ureter→5. bladder→6. urethral canal→7. forehead→8. trigeminal nerve→9. cerebellum and brain stem→10. neck and nape→11. nose→12. cerebrum→13. pituitary gland→14. esophagus and windpipe →15. parathyroid gland→16. thyroid gland→ 17. frontal sinus of other toes → 18. eye → 19. ear→20. trapezius muscle → 23. spleen→24. stomach →25. pancreas→26. duodenum→27. small intestine →28. transverse colon→ 29. descending colon→ 30. sigmoid colon and rectum → 31. anus → 32. genital gland →33. insomnia point → 34. point of checking diarrhea.

Medial surface of the left foot:

1. cervical vertebra →2. thoracic vertebra →3. lumbar vertebra→4. sacral vertebra→5. internal coccyx→6. uterus or prostate gland→7. internal rib→8. groin →9. lymph node in the lower body→10. medial hip joint→11. medial rectum and anus→12. medial sciatic nerve.

Lateral surface of the left foot:

1. shoulder →2. upper arm →3. elbow→4. knee→5. external coccyx→6. external genital gland→7. scapular bone→8. external rib →9. lymph node in the upper body→10. lateral hip joint→11. lower abdomen→12. lateral sciatic nerve.

Dorsum of the left foot:

1. upper jaw →2. lower jaw →3. tonsil→4. throat→5. thoracic lymph gland →6. windpipe→7. inner ear →8. chest and breast → 9. diaphragmatic muscle→10. ureter and deferent duct→11. lymph nodes in upper and lower body→12. Jiexi (ST 41).

Right foot   The sole of the right foot:

1. adrenal gland →2. celiac plexus →3. kidney→4. ureter→5. bladder→6. urethral canal (perineum)→7. forehead (frontal sinus) →8. trigeminal nerve→9. cerebellum and brain stem→10. neck and nape→11. nose→12. cerebrum→13. pituitary gland →14. esophagus and windpipe →15. parathyroid gland→ 16. thyroid gland→ 17. frontal

右足内侧：同左足内侧。

右足外侧：同左足外侧。

右足背：同左足背。

第二节 足部反射区具体定位、操作及适应证

为了加强反射区与人体相关器官的直接印象，就需要了解每个反射区同各器官的解剖比邻关系和生理结构，对记忆反射区的定位，有一定的辅助作用。当然要牢牢地掌握反射区的按摩就必需经常亲自动手去做，去体验，实践出真知。

【足底部心脏检查】

足底部检查一般都是从左足底心脏检查开始。目的有二：①了解被按摩者心脏情况，防止出现意外；②了解对方的敏感程度，以便调整术者的力度。

定位：左足第四、第五趾骨颈间为中心约拇指腹大小的范围。敏感点在该区偏上的部位。

手法：分轻、中、重三种。①轻：用右手拇指指腹由近至远从轻逐次稍加重推3次。正常情况无疼痛。②中：用右手弯曲的示指中节弧侧以中等手法逐次稍加重自近至远压刮3次，如出现疼痛，需关心对方的心功能情况。③重：以示指拳顶法压心脏反射区中心点，力度大于中手法。即使有疼痛感，也没有诊断意义。

sinus of other toes (head) → 18. eye → 19. ear →20. trapezius muscle→21. lung and bronchus→ 22. liver→ 23. gallbladder→ 24. stomach →25. pancreas →26. duodenum →27. small intestine → 28. cecum and appendix → 29. ileocecal valve → 30. ascending colon→ 31. transverse colon → 32. genital gland →33. insomnia point→ 34. point of checking diarrhea.

Medial surface of the right foot: the same as medial surface of the left foot.

Lateral surface of the right foot: the same as lateral surface of the left foot.

Dorsum of the left foot: the same as dorsum of the left foot.

Section 2 Foot Reflex Zones: Specific Location, Performance and Indications

In order to understand the direct relations between the reflex zones and their corresponding human organs, one needs to get to know the adjacent anatomical relations between each reflex zone and its corresponding organ, and the physiological structure of each reflex zone, which helps to memorize the location of reflex zones. Of course, to master the reflex zone massage firmly, one must frequently perform and experience it in person. As the old saying goes, "Practice makes perfect".

Heart Examination at the Sole of the Foot

Examination at the sole of foot generally starts from heart examination at the sole of the left foot for two purposes: ① getting to know the heart condition of the massaged to prevent accidents; ② getting to know the tenderness degree of the massaged so as to adjust the masseur's intensity of force.

Location: The range of the size of thumb pulp centering around the point between the forth and fifth toe bones. The tenderness point is situated at the upper region of the zone.

辅助手：始终用左手四个手指在足背相应位置反方向扶持。

注意点：检查手法，开始一定轻，均匀用力，并且逐次稍加重，尤其前1~6个按摩动作应该有相等的递增度，不应该不分轻重地多次按摩，失去反射区按摩的特点。按摩到5个动作后，一定要观察和询问对方的反应。

适应证：各种心脏病症和需要做足部反射区按摩的人。

【反射区定位、操作及适应证】

（一）足底各反射区

1. 肾上腺（图12、13）

定位：足底第二、第三跖骨颈之间，足掌人字形交叉点后方凹陷处。

手法：多用握足扣指法，以右手示指关节向骨缝缓慢顶入，出现酸胀感为佳，停留片刻再缓慢放松。逐次深入，直至出现微痛。一般按摩3~5次。

辅助手：扶持并协助，一要协助用力深入，二要不改变用力的方向。

注意点：①必须使右示指指节尖端直直顶入第二、第三骨骨缝间。②达到胀感后，要维持10~20秒后再缓缓放松。③以出现松解时的舒服感受为宜。④选位时

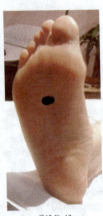

图12 Fig.12

Manipulations: They may be divided into three types, namely, lightness, moderateness and heaviness. ① lightness: Push with the finger pulp of the right thumb starting from the distal area, with gradually increasing force 3 times. There is no pain in normal situation. ② moderateness: Press-scrape with the hukou surface of the middle knuckle of the crooked index finger of the right hand in moderate manner progressively adding strength little by little from near to far for 3 times. If pain occurs, one needs to be concerned about the cardiac function of the massaged. ③ heaviness: Press the central point of the heart reflex zone by means of fist propping manipulation with the index finger, with more strength than moderate manipulation. Even there is sense of pain, there is no significance of diagnosis.

Supporting hand: Always support in the opposite direction at the dorsum of the foot with the four fingers of the left hand.

Cautionary notes: Check the manipulation to secure light stimulation at the very beginning and evenly exerting gradually increasing force. There should be equal gradient of increase especially for the first 1–6 massage movements. There should not be massage for many times with no difference of lightness and heaviness. After the 5th movement of massage, be sure to observe and inquire the reaction of the other side.

Indications: Those who suffer from all kinds of heart diseases and who need foot reflex zone massage.

Location, performance and indications of reflex zones

Ⅰ. Reflex Zones on the sole of Foot

1. Adrenal gland (Fig. 12, 13)

Location: The introcession posterior to the point of the intersection in lying "T" form on the sole, between the necks of the second and third metatarsal bones on the sole of the foot.

Manipulations: Gripping foot manipulation with buckling finger

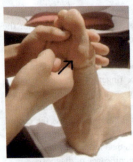

图13 Fig.13

要注意:顶入位差不多正对第三趾,掌握"宁外勿内,宁后勿前"的原则,再要注意足底的生理斜面。

适应证:与心脏、血管、血压、咳嗽、过敏、风湿关节痛、虚脱和性功能有关的病症均可。

2. 腹腔神经丛(太阳神经丛,图14、15)

定位:位于第二、第三跖骨近2/3处,肾反射区周围。

手法:用右手示指中节自远而近分侧作弧形压刮,自轻渐重各3~6次。

辅助手:在足背扶持给予反作用力。

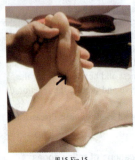

图15 Fig.15

注意点:①此反射区大致以肾为中心呈环形,压刮时可形成弧线。②逐渐加大,增加渗透感,动作要均匀。

适应证:腹胀、烦躁,缓解自主神经的紧张力及腹腔内各器官的病症。

is mostly used. Use the phalangeal joint of the index finger of right hand to prop into the bony suture slowly until soreness and distension occurs. Stay for a moment and then slowly relax the hold. Prop deeper and deeper time after time until slight pain occurs. Generally massage 3-5 times.

Supporting hand: Support and provide help. First, help the massaging hand to prop into forcefully. Second, do not change the direction of the force.

Cautionary notes: ① One must make the tip of the dorsal surface of the phalangeal joint of the index finger of the right hand straightly prop into the bony suture between the second and third metatarsal bones. ② When the massaged feels turgid, one should maintain 10-20 seconds and then slowly relax the hold. ③ It is appropriate to feel comfortable when force is released. ④ Be cautious about the position. The propping position should roughly opposite the third toe. Adhere to the principle of "Better lateral than medial, and better posterior than anterior". Moreover, pay attention to the physiological slant on the sole of the foot.

Indications: Diseases related to the heart, blood vessel, blood pressure, cough, allergy, rheumatic arthralgia, collapse and sexual function, etc.

2. celiac plexus (solar plexus, Fig. 14, 15)

Location: It is situated at the area across 2/3 palm of the foot, close to the second and third metatarsal bones, in the periphery of the kidney reflex zone.

Manipulations: Use the middle knuckle of the index finger of the right hand to scrape and press in arc form on the left and right side from far to

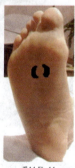

图14 Fig.14

3. 肾脏（图16、17）

定位：自肾上腺反射区向后延长1寸的范围。也可理解自脚掌人字缝尖向后延一指节。

手法：用示指中节自远至近均匀渗透压刮目3～6次，节奏要慢，力量要均匀。

辅助手：固定足背。

注意点：①肾区是足底部按摩中重要反射区，一要位置准，二要渗透均匀。②右手示指点中节全部压入再行刮压摩，均匀刮摩第一指节后再缓慢抬起为好。③避免压刮过程中变成示指近间关节着力，这将使被按摩者感受到不适，也不利于改善血液循环。

适应证：各种肾脏病和与肾有关的疾病。

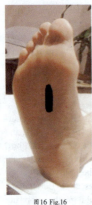

图16 Fig.16

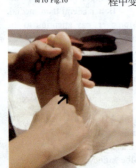

图17 Fig.17

near side, with gradually increasing force 3-6 times respectively.

Supporting hand: Support the dorsum of the foot by giving counteracting force.

Cautionary notes: ① This reflex zone centers around the zone to kidney and takes on circular form. Therefore, one may scrape and press in arc form. ② Progressively increase the strength and the sense of permeation with even movements.

Indications: Abdominal distension, restlessness, relief of the tension of vegetative nerve, and the diseases of the organs in abdominal cavity.

3. Kidney (Fig. 16, 17)

Location: The range extended 1 cun backward from the adrenal gland reflex zone, which may also be interpreted as the area extended 1 knuckle backward from the tip of the cleft in lying "T" form on the foot palm.

Manipulations: Use the middle knuckle of the index finger to scrape and press in evenly permeating manner from distal to local areas 3-6 times, with slow rhythm and even strength.

4. 输尿管（图18、19）

定位：从肾中开始先向后再斜向足底内侧的膀胱，是个贯通脚心的长形弧状条带区。

手法：用右手示指中节背面自肾中开始先压入到合适深度再向后压刮至离膀胱区约1/3的距离时，在不减轻压力的情况下，将右手内旋，边旋加压直到膀胱中点与示指中节背面近1/3相对，停留片刻慢慢抬起。如此从轻逐次加力压刮目3～6次。

辅助手：可以握足扣指法辅助，也可自然扶持足部或用拇指顶住按摩手，防止滑脱。

注意点：①此区在足底按摩中十分重要，做得好会明显提高效果。②自始至终强调均匀渗透，尤其下1/3段，如不按上法进行，很易走过场。③最后刮压到膀胱叫"到位"，不到位者，按摩质量不佳，也无需在膀胱处额外顶压。

适应证：对输尿管或泌尿系统疾病适用，对所有的足部反射区按摩者均应重点做，适用一切需排毒的疾患。

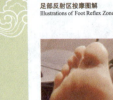

图18 Fig.18

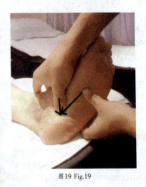

图19 Fig.19

4. Ureter (Fig. 18, 19)

Location: It is a long arc-form strip area that traverses the center of the sole, starting from the center of the kidney zone, going backward and then extending obliquely to the bladder zone on the medial surface of the sole of the foot.

Manipulations: Use the dorsal surface of the middle knuckle of the index finger of the right hand to press into the sole to a suitable depth starting from the center of the kidney zone, and then press-scrape backward until reaching the point about 1/3 from the bladder zone. Without reducing pressure, rotate the right hand inwards. While rotating, the masseur increases pressure until the center of the bladder zone opposites about 1/3 part of the dorsal surface of the middle knuckle of the right hand. Stay for a moment and slowly raise the hand. Press-scrape with gradually increasing force 3-6 times.

Supporting hand: Provide help by means of gripping foot manipulation with buckling finger, or naturally support the foot, or prop against the massaging hand with the thumb to prevent slip.

Cautionary notes: ① This zone is of vital importance in massage of the sole of the foot, and performing well will obviously enhance the effect. ② Emphasize evenness and permeation from the beginning to the end, especially the lower 1/3 segment. Not performing according to the above method will easily result in going through motions. ③ Scrap-pressing to the bladder zone at last is called "thorough". Being not thorough will lead to bad quality of massage. And there is no need to apply extra prop-pressing on the bladder zone.

Indications: Applicable to ureter or urinary system diseases. All the masseurs engaged in foot reflex zone massage should attach great importance to massage the zone, which is applied to all the disorders that need expelling toxins.

5. 膀胱（图20、21）

定位：足底内侧舟骨下方的软性稍突起处。在足跟内前方。

手法：用示指中节扇形压扭不过60°，稍有胀感即可。

辅助手：轻轻扶持足部，使其外展，以暴露足内侧的膀胱反射区，便于操作。

注意点：①该区较敏感，不需用大力，也不用旋转角度太大。②不要用示指扣拳法的关节尖顶压或砧孔状按压。

适应证：适用一切由上行感染引起的膀胱炎、尿道炎等。也可用于老年男性和老年女性的小便不利或小便不能控制等症状。

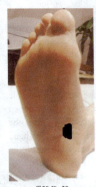

图20 Fig.20

6. 尿道（阴道或阴茎，图22、23）

定位：足内侧，自足跟内侧前方的膀胱反射区一直到内踝的后下方均属于该反射区。

手法：开始用拇指从膀胱后下方推向内踝的后下方，在推摩过程中靠近内下方时一定将手腕内旋，以拇指桡侧峰向内踝后下方的骨缝挤压，从而产生酸胀感为度。逐次加力3~6次。

辅助手：操作前先摸内踝后下方，以按

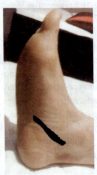

图22 Fig.22

5. Bladder (Fig. 20, 21)

Location: Soft slight enation inferior to the scaphoid bone on the medial surface of the sole of foot, medial anterior to the heel of foot.

Manipulations: Use the middle knuckle of the index finger to press-twist in a manner like a fan opening not more than 60°, until the patient. has a slight feeling of distension.

Supporting hand: Gently support the foot, making it stretch outward so as to expose the bladder reflex zone on the medial surface of the foot, convenient for performance.

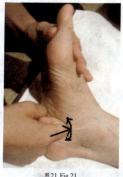

图21 Fig.21

Cautionary notes: ① The zone is relatively tender with no need of strong force and overly large angle of rotation. ② Do not use the tip of the phalangeal joint of the index finger in the buckling fist manipulation with index finger to prop-press or press like drilling.

Indications: All cystitis and urethritis induced by ascending infection, or symptoms of senile males' or females' dysuria or urinary incontinence.

6. Urinary canal (vagina or penis, Fig. 22, 23)

Location: On the medial surface of the foot, the area from the bladder reflex zone medial anterior to the heel all the way to the posterior inferior aspect of internal malleolus all belongs to the reflex zone.

Manipulations: At first use the thumb to push from posterior inferior aspect of bladder zone to posterior inferior aspect of the medial malleolus. During the course of push-rubbing, do rotate the

摩有的放矢。拇指推摩时，辅助手也可给予顶扶，防止滑脱。

注意点:本反射区须推至内踝后下方，获得麻胀感效果才佳。关键是通过扭手腕将拇指桡侧峰挤扣至骨缝中。

适应证：泌尿系感染、排尿障碍及一切会阴病症和性功能不佳者。

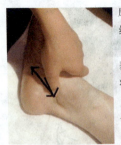

图23 Fig.23

7. 额窦（前额，图24、25）

定位：足踇趾顶端。

手法：用示指压刮和拇指推法均可。操作时先分开踇趾和第二趾，再行压刮3～6次。

辅助手：一定起到扶持踇趾或使第一、第二趾分开的作用。

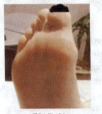

图24 Fig.24

注意点：①在压刮时，要想到踇趾顶端是圆的，不是平的，故要随着圆形顶端成弧形压刮才能使受力均匀。②如此逐渐加力时，患者则感到既舒服又到位。

适应证:前头痛、眼疾、视物不清、三叉神经痛和耳部疾患、额窦炎等。

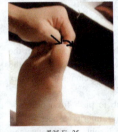

图25 Fig.25

wrist inwards when approaching the medial inferior aspect. Squeeze-press with the radial edge of the thumb toward the bony suture below the rear of the medial malleolus until soreness and distension occurs. Progressively increase the force 3-6 times.

Supporting hand: Before the operation, first touch the posterior inferior aspect of medial malleolus, making the massage have a definite object in view. When push-rubbing with the thumb, the supporting hand may also prop and support to prevent from slip.

Cautionary notes: For this reflex zone, be sure to pushing the posterior inferior aspect of medial malleolus until the best effect of feeling numb and distension. The key point is to make the radial edge of thumb squeeze into the bony suture by wringing the wrist.

Indications: those who suffer from urinary system infection, urinary hindrance, all perineal diseases, and sexual dysfunction.

7. Frontal sinus (forehead, Fig. 24, 25)

Location: On the tip of the big toe.

Manipulations: Both the pressing and scraping manipulation with the index finger and the pushing manipulation with the thumb will do. When performing, first the masseur separates the big toe from the second toe, and then he presses and scrapes 3-6 times.

Supporting hand: Be sure to function supporting the thumb toe or separating the first toe from the second toe.

Cautionary notes: ① When scraping and pressing, take into account that the tip of the big toe is round not flat. Therefore, only by scraping and pressing in arc form along with the round tip can one make the force received evenly. ② If the masseur gradually increases the force like that, the patient will feel comfortable and thorough.

Indications: Forehead pain, disease of the eyes, blurred vision, trigeminal neuralgia, disorders of ears, frontal sinusitis, etc.

8. 三叉神经（图26、27）

定位： 在大踇趾末节外侧的中上段，远端与额窦反射区外侧重叠，在趾甲侧面的远侧1/2处，为上支。沿此向踇趾的外下方的隆起部为中支，再从踇趾外侧向近端为下支。

手法： 用拇指指端着力扣点额窦的外侧拇指甲远侧1/2处，产生痛感为度为上支；边扣边向踇趾外下推压约1厘米左右，产生酸痛感为中支；拇指端退回原处，再以扣指法向踇趾外侧压推，产生痛感为下支。根据患者耐受情况施力，重复2～4遍。

辅助手： 固定被按摩的足。

注意点： ①此反射区难做，必须按以上要领才能获得成功；②此反射区最敏感，大部分都痛，要手下留情，逐次加力，并了解对方的反映，否则费力不讨好，或者做不到位。

适应证： 头痛、面神经麻痹、三叉神经痛、牙痛、头部侧面及五官科的病痛。

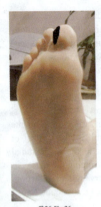

图26 Fig.26

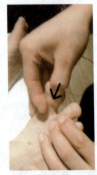

图27 Fig.27

8. Trigeminal nerves (Fig. 26, 27)

Location: At the middle superior segment of the medial surface of the end knuckle of the big toe. The distal end overlaps the lateral aspect of frontal sinus reflex zone. The superior branch refers to the area 1/2 distally from the lateral surface of toenail. The middle branch refers to the area from the superior branch to protuberant portion of lateral inferior aspect of the big toe. The inferior branch refers to area from the lateral surface of the big toe to the proximal end.

Manipulations: Digital-press forcefully with the tip of the thumb the area 1/2 distally from the big toe nail, outside the frontal sinus, and bring about the feeling of pain, which is called the superior branch. While digging, the masseur pushes and presses about 1 cm toward the lateral inferior aspect of the big toe, and cause the feeling of sourness and pain, which is called middle branch. Let the tip of the thumb return to the original place, and then push and press toward the lateral aspect of thumb toe by using buckling finger manipulation, and bring about the feeling of pain, which is called inferior branch. Exert force according to the patient's tolerance of strength, and repeat 2-4 times.

Supporting hand: Fix the massaged foot.

Cautionary notes: ① It is difficult to perform massage at this reflex zone. Only by doing according to the above-mentioned essentials can one become successful; ② This reflex zone is the most tender one, most portion of which feels ached. Therefore, one should perform mercifully by increasing force progressively and minding the reaction of the other side. Or else one will do a hard but thankless job or not perform thoroughly.

Indications: Headache, facial paralysis, trigeminal neuralgia, toothache, and diseases of the lateral surface of head and five sensory organs.

9. 小脑和脑干（图28、29）

定位：位于踇趾趾腹外下部，下界不超过趾间关节，也不能在踇趾的外侧面上。

手法：用示指拳顶法和捏指法均可，从轻逐渐加力按压3~6次。

辅助手：用示指拳顶法时辅助手应该在踇趾背侧扶持。

注意点：①由于平面图不易将踇趾趾腹与趾间关节横纹显示清楚，故不要错误地将小脑反射区定在踇趾趾间横纹以下，更不要定在踇趾近节趾骨外侧面；②小脑和脑干反射区应该以按摩手和辅助手相互挤压，才能获得适度的刺激量。

适应证：运动平衡失调、多动症和晕眩等症。

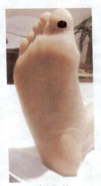

图28 Fig.28

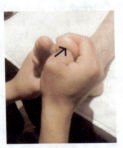

图29 Fig.29

10. 颈项（图30、31）

定位：位于踇趾根横纹处。有两个敏感点，分别位于趾根两侧。

手法：以拇指指端扣法，边扣边由外向内移，在趾根下方外侧和内侧，触到滚动条状物，同时感到胀痛，由轻逐渐加力，反复3~4。

9. Cerebellum and brainstem (Fig. 28, 29)

Location: In the lateral inferior aspect of the finger pulp of the big toe, with the lower bound neither surpassing the phalangeal joint of the toe, nor on the lateral surface of the big toe.

Manipulations: Both the fist propping manipulation with the index finger and the nipping finger manipulation will do. Press with gradually increasing force 3-6 times.

Supporting hand: When fist propping manipulation with the index finger is in use, the supporting hand should support the dorsal surface of the big toe.

Cautionary notes: ① It is not easy for the plan view picture to clearly display the finger pulp of the big toe and the cross striation of the interphalangeal joint of the big toe. Therefore, neither mistakenly locate the cerebellum reflex zone below the cross striation of the interphalangeal joint of the big toe, nor locate it on the lateral surface of proximal phalanx of the big toe; ② For the reflex zones to cerebellum and brainstem, the massaging hand and the supporting hand should mutually squeeze and press, so as to achieve moderate amount of stimulation.

Indications: Kinetic dysequilibrium, minimal brain dysfunction, and vertigo, etc.

10. Neck and nape (Fig. 30, 31)

Location: Situated at the cross striation of the root of big toe. There are two tender points, situated at the two sides of the root of toe respectively.

Manipulations: By using buckling manipulation with the finger tip of thumb, the masseur moves the tip of thumb from outside to inside while buckling. On the lateral and medial surfaces below the root of toe, the masseur touches a rolling bar-shape stuff, and meanwhile, the patient feels distending and ache. Then the masseur

辅助手：只需扶脚即可。

注意点：①按摩者的拇指尖必须从踇趾的外侧开始扣紧；②在内侧边扣边旋扭时，不能放松，尤其在两侧趾根处；③如果敏感点不清楚时，可将旋扭的度数加大到180度。

适应证：落枕、颈项各部痛症和由颈部引起的其他头痛、颈椎不适、胸背不适等。

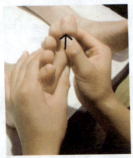

图31 Fig.31

11. 鼻（图32、33）

定位：踇趾末节的内侧。

手法：用示指拳顶法，正对踇趾末节内侧的凹陷处，逐次加力，一般3～5次。最后一次时间较长，并持续片刻再缓慢放松，此称"通气法"。

辅助手：必须以辅助的拇、示指固定援脚的踇趾和脚。

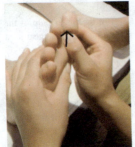

图33 Fig.33

注意点：做"通气法"时，因为末节趾骨的凹面向远端倾斜，故应将手腕抬高，才能正对鼻的反射区凹陷处。

适应证：各种鼻部疾病患、呼吸道疾患和面部五官病痛。

increases the force progressively from light degree, repeating 3-4 times.

Supporting hand: Supporting the foot is ok.

Cautionary notes: ① The masseur must buckle the finger tip of the thumb tightly just from the lateral surface of the big toe; ② When rotating while buckling on the medial surface of the thumb toe, the masseur cannot relax the hold, especially on the two sides of the root of toe; ③ If the tenderness point is not clear, increase the degree of rotation to 180.

Indications: Stiff neck, neck pain, and other headache, indisposition of cervical vertebra and chest-back, induced by cervical problems.

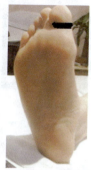

图 30 Fig.30

11. Nose (Fig. 32, 33)

Location: Situated at the medial surface of the paratelum of the big toe.

Manipulations: Apply the fist propping manipulation with the index finger and progressively increase the force generally for 3-5 times, facing the introcession on the medial surface of the paratelum of the big toe. The last propping takes longer time and should be kept on for a moment and slowly relax, which is called "connecting qi method".

Supporting hand: Be sure to use the auxiliary thumb and index finger to fix the big toe and the foot.

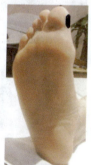

图 32 Fig.32

12. 大脑（图34、35）

定位：跚趾趾腹的全部区域均属于大脑反射区。

手法：用示指中节背面从轻逐次加重压刮，将大跚趾分成三条纵线各压3次以上。

辅助手：在足背面扶持，保证反作用力。

注意点：①大脑功能非常复杂，不要遗漏；②两手配合使压刮的力度适中；③必要时可增拇指、示指的捏揉动作。

适应证：头痛、失眠、脑部疾病、头晕、脑胀、高血压及全身的功能紊乱性疾病。

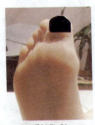

图34 Fig.34

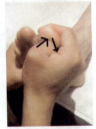

图35 Fig.35

13. 脑垂体（图36、37）

定位：位于跚趾趾腹的中央深部。

手法：用示指拳顶法的指关节外侧按压，逐次加力，最后一次要延长按压时间。

辅助手：示、中指在跚趾背侧扶持，拇指协助加力。

注意点：①用示指关节外侧按压，目的是按触面积小，容易压入深层；②辅助

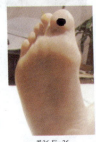

图36 Fig.36

Cautionary notes: When applying "connecting qi method", one should raise the wrist, so as to face the introcession of the nose reflex zone, for the introcession surface of the paratelum of the thumb toe slants toward the distal end.

Indications: All kinds of nasal diseases, respiratory tract diseases, and disorders of five sensory organs on the face.

12. Cerebrum (Fig. 34, 35)

Location: All the area of the finger pulp of the thumb toe belongs to the cerebrum reflex zone.

Manipulations: Scrape and press with gradually increasing force using the dorsal surface of the middle knuckle of the index finger. Divide the thumb toe into three vertical lines and press them over 3 times respectively.

Supporting hand: Support the dorsum of the foot, ensuring counteracting force.

Cautionary notes : ① The function of the cerebrum is very complex, so do not omit something by mistake; ② make the intensity of the strength of scraping and pressing moderate by combining the two hands; ③ If necessary, the kneading and rubbing movements of thumb and index finger may be added.

Indications: Headache, insomnia, encephalopathy, dizziness, cerebral distention, hypertension and functional disorder all over the body, etc.

13. Pituitary gland (Fig. 36, 37)

Location: Situated at the deep place in the center of the finger pulp of the big toe.

Manipulations: Use the lateral surface of the phalangeal joint in the fist propping manipulation with the index finger to press, and increase the force progressively. The last pressing requires prolonging

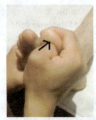

图37 Fig.37

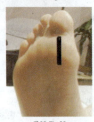

图38 Fig.38

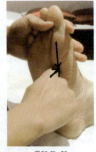

图39 Fig.39

手有两个作用,一是保持按压的部位不移动,二是掌握压入的稳定过程,不会突然太重。

适应证:全身内分泌功能失调、各内分泌腺的不足或亢进、妇女围绝经期综合征、小儿发育迟缓及抗衰老等。

14. 食管和气管(图38、39)

定位:第一跖趾关节偏内侧的纵向带状区。

手法:用示指扣拳法的示指关节向内倾斜向近端压刮,着力点主要在第一跖趾关节的内侧。越偏内侧,越易出现敏感带。

辅助手:需将第一跖趾关节背侧把住,使两手的合力产生对第一跖趾关节足底内侧的压力。

注意点:①食管和气管在双足都有,其敏感部位在第一跖趾关节足底的内侧,上连颈部,下连胃部和肺及支气管;②辅助手和按摩手同时用力,避免将踇趾搬向背侧。

适应证:食管和气管的各种病症、胃部和肺及支气管的病症等。

the time of pressing.

Supporting hand: Support the dorsal surface of the big toe with the index and middle fingers, the thumb used to help increase the force.

Cautionary notes: ① Use the lateral surface of the phalangeal joint of the index finger to press in order to reduce the touching area and be liable to press into the deeper layer. ② There are two functions for the supporting hand. One is to keep the pressing region from removing, the other is to control the steady course of pressing, avoiding sudden heaviness.

Indications: General endocrine disorder, deficiency or accentuation of endocrine glands, climacteric syndrome of women, retarded development of children and anti-aging, etc.

14. Esophagus and windpipe (Fig. 38, 39)

Location: At the vertical strip area inclined to the medial surface of the first metatarsophalangeal joint.

Manipulations: Applying the buckling fist manipulation with the index finger, the masseur uses the phalangeal joint of the index finger to press-scrape toward the proximal end by making the joint slanting inward. The point at which the force is given is mainly situated at the medial surface of the first metatarsophalangeal joint. The more medially inclined, the easier the occurrence of tenderness strip area.

Supporting hand: Be sure to tightly hold the dorsal surface of the first metatarsophalangeal joint, making resultant of forces from the two hands form the pressure against the medial surface of the sole of the first metatarsophalangeal joint.

Cautionary notes: ① The reflex zones to esophagus and windpipe are situated at two feet, and the tenderness regions of them are situated at the he medial surface of the sole of the first

15. 甲状旁腺（图40、41）

定位：位于第一跖趾关节外侧的远侧，靠近跚趾根横纹附近。

手法：用拇指指端顶压法，或用示指中节顶压法。

辅助手：双手抱脚，小趾侧的拇、示指将足跚趾向远侧牵拉，同时跚趾侧的拇指尖端由外向内横向顶住第一跖趾关节远侧跚趾横纹处，牵跚趾的手松开，另一手继续顶压，此时则出现麻胀感。如此重复3次，并逐次加力。也可用示指中节顶压第一跖趾关节处。

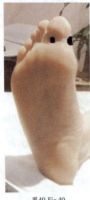

图40 Fig.40

注意点：①必须按上述要领才能做出麻胀的感觉来，要注意按摩手拇指尖的顶压方向。②第一跖趾关节的内侧也可用拇指揉法。

适应证：甲状旁腺功能异常引起的缺钙、筋骨酸痛、抽筋、手足痉挛、指甲病、白内障等。

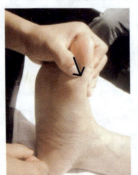

图41 Fig.41

metatarsophalangeal joint, connecting the neck upward, and the stomach, lung and bronchus downward. ② The supporting hand and the massaging hand should exert force simultaneously, avoiding pulling the big toe toward the dorsal surface.

Indications: Various diseases of the esophagus and windpipe as well as diseases of the stomach, lung and bronchus.

15. Parathyroid gland (Fig. 40, 41)

Location: Situated at the area distally away from the lateral aspect of the first metatarsophalangeal joint, approaching the vicinity of the cross striation of the big toe.

Manipulations: Apply prop-pressing manipulation with the tip of thumb or prop-pressing manipulation with the middle knuckle of the index finger.

Supporting hand: Hold the foot in two hands, with the thumb and the index finger beside the little toe dragging the big toe of the foot distally, and meanwhile, the tip of the big toe transversely propping from outside to inside against the cross striation of the big toe, which is distally apart from the lateral surface of the first metatarsophalangeal joint. Release the hand that drags the big toe, with the other hand continuing propping and pressing. At this time the sense of numbness and distension occurs. Repeat like that for 3 times, and progressively increase the force. Or use the middle knuckle of the index finger to prop and press the first metatarsophalangeal joint.

Cautionary notes: ① Be sure to perform in line with the above-mentioned essentials so as to get the feeling of numbness and turgidity. Pay attention to the direction of the propping and pressing given by the tip of the thumb of the massaging hand. ② The kneading manipulation with the thumb may be applied to the medial surface of first metatarsophalangeal joint.

Indications: Calcium deficiency, aching pain of bones and

16. 甲状腺（图42、43）

定位：足底第一跖趾关节周围与第二跖骨之间的区域。

手法：用示指间关节压刮法。

辅助手：扶持足背中部。

注意点：①对甲状腺反射区的概念应形成新的概念，即第一跖趾关节附近都属于甲状腺反射区。②无论何种手法只要做出感觉即可。

适应证：甲状腺功能异常、失眠、心悸、情绪不佳、肥胖和消瘦等。

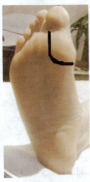

图42 Fig.42

17. 额窦（图44、45）

定位：第二至第五趾关节膨大部分。

手法：以示指压刮法自远而近，从轻逐渐加力各压刮3~6次，再以毛巾包住各趾，用拇示指顺时针和逆时针各捏揉3~6遍。

辅助手：在做压刮时，辅助手需固定各趾背侧；包住脚趾捏揉时，两手都已成为按摩手了。

注意点：①压刮时要求将各趾关节膨大部位都刮到，不要遗漏，同时注意不要因刮得过长而顶痛膨大以近中节或近节趾的底面。②包巾捏揉时用力要均匀。

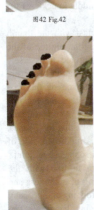

图44 Fig.44

muscles, muscle cramps, carpopedal spasm, fingernail disease and cataract, etc. induced by disfunction of parathyroid gland.

16. Thyroid gland (Fig. 42, 43)

Location: The area between the periphery of the first metatarsophalangeal joint of the sole and the second metatarsal bone.

Manipulations: Apply the pressing and scraping manipulation with the interphalangeal joint of the index finger.

Supporting hand: Supporting the central part in the dorsum of the foot.

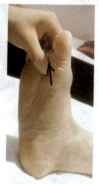

图43 Fig.43

Cautionary notes: ① To the concept of the thyroid gland reflex zone, one should have new concept, i.e., the vicinity of the first metatarsophalangeal joint all belongs to the thyroid gland reflex zone. ② Whatever manipulation is applied, occurrence of feeling is ok.

Indications: Dysfunction of thyroid gland, insomnia, palpitations, blue mood, obesity and emaciation.

17. Frontal sinus (Fig. 44, 45)

Location: Most part of the dilation of phalangeal joints of the 2nd to 5th toes.

Manipulations: Apply the pressing and scraping manipulation with the index finger to press and scrape from distal to local areas, progressively increasing the force 3-6 times respectively, and then wrap these toes with towel, kneading with the thumb and index finger clockwise and anticlockwise 3-6 times respectively.

Supporting hand: When pressing and scraping, the assistant should fix the dorsal surfaces of these toes; When kneading by

适应证：各种头部疾患及五官的各种病症以及失眠、眩晕等症。

18. 眼（图46、47）

定位：第二、第三趾中近节的底面和两个侧面，趾根两侧与足底面的斜角处为眼的敏感点，在第二、第三趾背侧的趾足间也有一个敏感点。

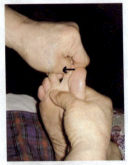

图45 Fig.45

手法：用拇指指尖捏掐趾根敏感点，每次由轻渐重或捏3次，再用拇指指腹由远而近推摩每个足趾的内、下、外三个面，最后再用拇指侧峰按压第二、第三趾根背侧的敏感点3次。

辅助手：辅助手从足背扶持住各趾。

注意点：①拇指尖捏掐时，一定要在趾根的底部和内外侧交角处才行。②在用拇指指腹推摩内外侧时，最好斜向足背侧，避免指甲顶伤足趾根部。③如果足趾太短，可横向推摩。

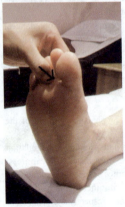

图47 Fig.47

wrapping the toes, the two hands have become the massaging hand.

Cautionary notes: ① When scraping and pressing, the masseur is required to reach the dilation region of the phalangeal joints of the toes without omission. Meanwhile, the masseur should pay attention not to scrape so long as to cause pain by propping against the dilation and the undersurface of the middle and proximal phalangeal joints of the toes. ② The masseur should exert force evenly when kneading by wrapping with towel.

Indications: All kinds of head diseases, the disorders of five sensory organs, insomnia and vertigo, etc.

18. Eyes (Fig. 46, 47)

Location: On the undersurface and the two lateral surface of the middle and proximal knuckles of the second and third toes. Two sides of the root of the toe and the oblique angle of the planta surface are the tenderness points of the eyes. There is still a tenderness point between the phalanxes on the dorsal surfaces of the second and third toes.

Manipulations: Nip the tenderness point at the root of the toe with the tip of the thumb, each time gradually from light to heavy or nipping for 3 times. Then push-rub the medial, inferior and lateral surfaces of each toe with the finger pulp of thumb from distal to local areas. Last but not least, press with the lateral edge of the thumb the tenderness points on the dorsal surfaces of roots of the second and third toes 3 times.

Supporting hand: Support each toe from the dorsum of the foot.

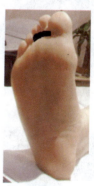

图46 Fig.46

Cautionary notes: ① When nipping

适应证：各种眼部疾病及与肝脏有关的病症。

19. 耳（图48、49）

定位：第四、第五趾中节两趾的底面和内外侧，每个趾根部两侧和第四、第五趾根间背侧的趾蹼处都有5个敏感点。

手法：手法与眼相同。

辅助手：示指拳顶时，需用辅助手在足背的趾背侧辅助。

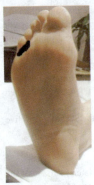

图48 Fig.48

注意点：①小趾的敏感点有变化，小趾内侧的敏感点应在外侧趾根处随着脚趾的变形而移到了小趾的足正中间。②有足癣的人，事先应涂脚气膏，再做操作。

适应证：一切耳部疾患和肾功能不佳者均可。

20. 斜方肌（图50、51）

定位：足底脚掌前半部、眼耳反射区后方，呈横向带状区。

手法：用示指扣拳法的示指中节从外向内压刮3～6次。

辅助手：将各趾扒成微屈状，使脚掌放松。

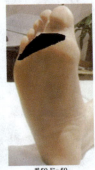

图50 Fig.50

with the thumb, be sure to perform at the bottom of the root of toe and the crossing angle of medial and lateral surface. ② When pushing and rubbing medial and lateral surfaces, it is suggestible to perform obliquely toward the dorsum of the foot, so as to prevent the finger nail from injuring the root of toe by propping. ③ Transversely push-rubbing is allowed if the toes are too short.

Indications: All kinds of eyes diseases and the disorders related to the liver.

19. Ear (Fig. 48, 49)

Location: The undersurface and the medial lateral surface of the two middle knuckles of the fourth and fifth toes. There are 5 tenderness points situated at the two sides of the roots of each toe, and the toe web between the dorsal surfaces of the fourth and fifth toes.

Manipulation: The same as that of eyes.

Supporting hand: When fist propping manipulation with the index finger is used, it is necessary for the supporting hand to provide help on the dorsal surface of the toe from the dorsum of foot.

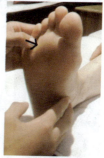

图49 Fig.49

Cautionary notes: ① There is little change for the tenderness point on the little toe. The tenderness point on the medial surface should be situated at the lateral root of toe, and will move to right middle of the little toe. ② For the patient with tinea pedis, it is required to apply beriberi ointment in advance, and then perform.

Indications: All the ear diseases and renal conditions.

20. Trapezius muscle (Fig. 50,51)

Location: At front half of the sole of foot, posterior to the reflex

注意点：①辅助手用力将各足趾挡住，不能翘趾。②脚底厚者可用按摩棒。

适应证：落枕、颈背酸痛、肩臂不适等症。

21. 肺和支气管（图52、53）

定位：脚掌后半部分，斜方肌的后方，内界是甲状腺，构成横向带状区。

手法：与斜方肌相同，只是位置偏后方。操作时肺用示指钩拳法；支气管用双拇示推摩法。

辅助手：扒住脚的各趾，使其微屈、放松。

注意点：要使脚掌放松，操作时如果脚掌太厚也可用按摩棒。

适应证：肺部和气管、支气管的各种病症。如：呼吸道感染、哮喘、胸闷等。

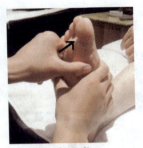

图51 Fig.51

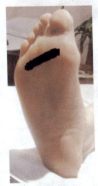

图52 Fig.52

zones to eyes and ears, taking on transverse strip area.

Manipulation: Use the middle knuckle of the index finger in the hooking fist manipulation with index finger to scrape and press from outside to inside for 3-6 times.

Supporting hand: Push the toes aside in subtly bending form, making the palm of foot relax.

Cautionary notes: ① The supporting hand firmly holds out against the toes so as to prevent the toes from tilting. ② For patient with thick foot plate, massage club may be used.

Indications: Stiff neck, aching pain of nape, discomfort of shoulder and back, etc.

21. Lung and bronchus (Fig. 52, 53)

Location: At the second half of the palm of foot, in the rear of trapezius muscle, with the medial bound being thyroid gland, forming transverse strip area.

Manipulation: The same as that of trapezius muscle, with the position inclined to the rear. Apply hooking manipulation with the index finger when performing. For bronchus, apply push-rubbing manipulation with the double thumbs.

Supporting hand: Hold on to the toes making them subtly bend and relax.

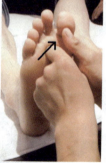

图53 Fig.53

Cautionary notes: Make the palm of foot relax. When performing, massage stick may be used if the palm of foot is too thick.

Indications: All kinds of diseases of lung, trachea, and bronchus, such as respiratory tract infection, asthma and chest distress, etc.

22. 心脏（图54、55）

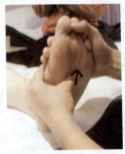

图55 Fig.55

定位：中心点在左脚第四、第五跖骨颈之间，上界被肺覆盖，下界与脾相邻。敏感点在肺覆盖的部位。

手法：摸好中心，用示指拳顶法，顶压力3～6次，逐渐加力，并延长时间。

辅助手：需在足背部扶持，起反作用力。

注意点：①顶压时，不要使用任何移动手法，如扭转、压刮等。②对有急性心脏病发作患者，手法要轻。

适应证：各种心脏功能紊乱性疾病，如心律不齐，气短、胸闷、易疲劳、睡眠不好、多梦等。

23. 脾（图56、57）

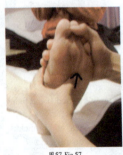

图57 Fig.57

定位：左脚第四、第五跖骨基底间，心反射区下方。

手法：用示指拳顶法，逐次加重顶压3～6次。

辅助手：在足背部扶持，起反作用力。

注意点：用示指顶按，不要有压刮法。

22. Heart (Fig. 54, 55)

Location: The central point is situated between necks of the fourth and fifth metatarsal bones of right foot, with the upper bound covered by lung reflex zone and lower bound connected with spleen reflex zone. The tender point is in the region covered by lung reflex zone.

Manipulation: Grope to reach the central point. Using fist propping manipulation to with index finger, prop and press for 3-6 times by increasing force progressively and prolonging time.

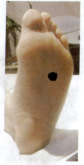

图54 Fig.54

Supporting hand: It is necessary to support the dorsum of foot, forming counteracting force.

Cautionary notes: ① When prop-pressing, do not apply any manipulation that causes moving, such as torsion, scraping and pressing. ② Apply gentle manipulation for the patient with acute heart disease attack.

Indications: All kinds of cardiac dysfunction diseases such as irregularity of heart rate, shortness of breath, chest distress, fatigue, poor sleep, dreaminess.

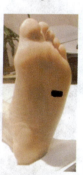

23. Spleen (Fig. 56, 57)

图56 Fig.56

Location: Between the basal parts of the fourth and fifth metatarsal bones, inferior to the heart reflex zone.

Manipulation: Using fist propping manipulation with index finger, the masseur props and presses progressively by increasing the strength for 3-6 times.

适应证：贫血、免疫功能低下引起的病症、炎症、发热、皮肤过敏，消化不良及肿瘤患者化疗时引起的不适等。

24. 肝（图58、59）

定位：右脚第四、第五跖骨足底面，上界与肺反射区重叠。

手法：用示指中节横向自远而近压刮，逐渐加力，反复3~6次。

辅助手：有效地挡住右足背的部位。

注意点：①肝区上界与肺重叠，下界与肠相交。②为使按摩有效，可用右手的示指扣拳法自远而近压刮。③辅助手一定要用力挡住。

适应证：各种肝脏疾患，如肝炎、肝肿大、中毒症、烟酒过量以及肝火旺盛引起的焦躁不安、食欲不佳、睡眠异常等。

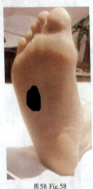

图58 Fig.58

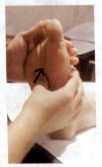

图59 Fig.59

Supporting hand: Support the dorsum of foot, forming counteracting force.

Cautionary notes: Prop and press with index finger instead of using scraping and pressing method.

Indications: Diseases induced by anemia, immunologic function deficiency, inflammation, fever, dermal allergy, indigestion, and discomfort caused by chemical therapy for tumor patient.

24. Liver (Fig. 58, 59)

Location: On the undersurface of the fourth and fifth metatarsal bones of right foot, with the upper bound overlapping the lung reflex zone.

Manipulation: Press and scrape with the middle knuckle of index finger transversely from distal to local areas by increasing force progressively 3-6 times repeatedly.

Supporting hand: Hold out against the dorsum of foot effectively.

Cautionary notes: ① The upper bound of liver zone overlaps lung zone, and the lower bound of liver overlaps intestine zone. ② In order to make the massage effective, buckling fist manipulation with index finger of right hand may be used to press and scrape from distal to local areas. ③ The supporting hand must hold out against the dorsum of foot forcefully.

Indications: All kinds of liver diseases such as hepatitis, hepatomegaly, toxipathy, restlessness, poor appetite and sleep disorder induced by over drinking and smoking, and hyperactivity of liver-fire.

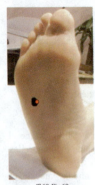

图60 Fig.60

25. 胆囊（图60红点）

定位：右脚掌第三、第四跖骨上部肝反射区内。

手法：示指拳顶法，斜向外上方顶压3～4次。

辅助手：需有效地在足背扶持用力。

注意点：①此反射区部位深，需用示指背节尖部顶入。②也可用器具顶压，先向第三、第四跖骨间顶压，得气后再将棒尖向外顶压出现痛感为佳。

适应证：胆囊疾患，如胆囊炎、胆结石。胆道疾患如剑突下疼痛、消化不良、腹胀、大便干等。

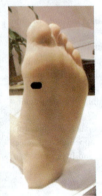

图61 Fig.61

26. 胃（图61、62）

定位：第一跖骨趾关节后方的甲状腺反射区之后，敏感点在第一跖骨的内侧缘。

手法：示指拳顶法，从轻到重顶压3～6次。

辅助手：在足背扶持，起反作用力。

注意点：①胃反射区位于第一跖骨体部，可以稍用力顶压，和胰比较，敏感度稍差。②对于有胃痛症状的患者，必须将顶压点重点向第一跖骨内侧移，才有效。③胃部不适

25. Gallbladder (the red point in Fig. 60)

Location: In the liver reflex zone superior to the third and fourth metatarsal bones of the right foot palm.

Manipulation: Applying fist propping manipulation with index finger, the masseur prop-presses obliquely outward for 3-4 times.

Supporting hand: It is necessary to effectively support the dorsum of right foot.

Cautionary notes: ① The reflex zone is situated deeper, requiring the tip of the dorsal knuckle to prop into. ② Or prop and press with equipment. First prop and press toward the third and fourth metatarsal bones. After acu-esthesia, make the tip of the club prop and press outward until feeling of pain occurs.

Indications: Diseases of gallbladder, such as cholecystitis and gallstone, and disorders of biliary tract, such as subxiphoid pain, indigestion, abdominal distention and dry stools.

26. Stomach (Fig. 61, 62)

Location: Posterior to the thyroid gland reflex zone which is posterior to the phalangeal joint of the first metatarsal bone, with the tender point at the medial border of the first metatarsal bone.

Manipulation: Using fist propping manipulation with index finger, the masseur props and presses with gradually increasing force 3-6 times.

Supporting hand: Support the dorsum of foot, forming counteracting force.

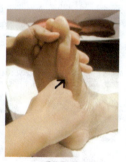

图62 Fig.62

的患者，应多在此区按摩。

适应证：各种胃部疾患，如胃炎、胃溃疡、胃肠功能紊乱、胃下垂等。

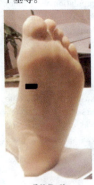

图63 Fig.63

27. 胰（图63）

定位：位于第一跖骨靠近基底部的部位，远侧是胃反射区，近侧是十二指肠反射区。

手法：同胃反射区的按摩手法，但比胃反射区的手法稍轻。

辅助手：同胃部的方法。

注意点：①因为胰反射区接近第一跖骨的基底部的骨骼突起，故用力稍轻。②辅助手也应同时用力。

适应证：胰本身的疾病，如胰腺炎、胰腺癌、糖尿病，还有消化系统疾病及其他症状。

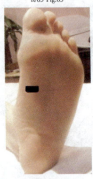

图64 Fig.64

28. 十二指肠（图64）

定位：位于第一跖骨基底和与楔骨形成的关节线上。

手法：用示指拳顶法顶压法。

辅助手：同前。

注意点：①十二指肠反射区很易出现疼痛，一是不要太重，让对方能忍受，同时也

Cautionary notes: ① The stomach reflex zone is situated at the region of the first metatarsal bone, which allows propping and pressing with slight force. Compared with the spleen zone, the sensitivity is low. ② For the patient with gastralgia symptoms, be sure to move the important point of propping and press toward the medial aspect of the metatarsal bone, so as to be effective. ③ For the patient with stomach discomfort, it is necessary to massage this zone more often.

Indications: All kinds of diseases of stomach such as gastritis, gastric ulcer, gastrointestinal disturbance and gastroptosia.

27. Pancreas (Fig. 63)

Location: Situated at the region close to the basal part of the first metatarsal bone. The distal area is the stomach reflex zone, and the proximal area is the duodenum reflex zone.

Manipulation: The same as the massage manipulation of the stomach reflex zone, but a little lighter that manipulation.

Supporting hand: The same as the method for stomach.

Cautionary notes: ① Because the pancreas reflex zone approaches the skeleton enation of the basal part of the first metatarsal bone, it is necessary to exert force a little bit lightly. ② The supporting hand should exert force simultaneously.

Indications: Diseases of pancreas, such as pancreatitis, pancreatic cancer, diabetes, and disease of digestive system and other symptoms.

28. Duodenum (Fig. 64)

Location: Situated at the joint line formed by the base of the first metatarsal bone and the cuneiform bone.

Manipulation: Apply the propping and pressing method of fist propping manipulation with index finger.

要给予适当的刺激，此反射区是一个重点保健穴位；②在同时压刮胃、胰、十二指肠时也要尽量做得均匀些。

适应证：胃和十二指肠的疾病，如胃炎、十二指肠炎、胃溃疡、十二指肠溃疡等。

29. 小肠（图65、66）

定位：除脚掌和脚后跟，大部分脚心的部位都是小肠的反射区。

手法：四指屈曲，以第二至第五指的近指节关节着力，有节奏地压刮10次左右，常出现热感。

辅助手：扶持足背中部，使足部稳固。

注意点：①小肠反射区定位宜宽广些才符合它在腹腔内占有的位置。②有节奏地多次压刮，可使脚心发热，同时也促进了胃肠蠕动。③如按摩师的手较大，可用三个指关节也可。④有怕痒的人，一摸脚心就痒，此时可先不用移动手法。

适应证：消化吸收不正常的病症，如腹胀、食后排空慢等。

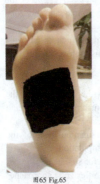

图65 Fig.65

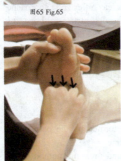

图66 Fig.66

Supporting hand: Ditto.

Cautionary notes: ① Pain easily occurs in the duodenum reflex zone. Therefore, do not perform too heavily so as to make the other person be able to tolerate, and meanwhile, giving proper stimulus. This reflex zone is a key acupoint for health care. ② When press and scrape the reflex zones to stomach, pancreas and duodenum simultaneously, perform as evenly as possible.

Indications: Diseases of stomach and duodenum, such as gastritis, duodenitis, gastric ulcer and duodenal ulcer.

29. Small intestine (Fig. 65, 66)

Location: Except the palm of foot and the heel, most region of the center of foot belongs to the small intestine reflex zone.

Manipulation: Flex the four fingers, give force with the proximal phalangeal joints of the second to fifth fingers, and press and scrape rhythmically about 10 times. Under such circumstance, the patient often feel hot.

Supporting hand: Support the central part of dorsum of foot, making the foot steady and firm.

Cautionary notes: ① The location of the small intestine reflex zone should be broad so as to conform to its corresponding position in abdominal cavity. ② Scrape and press rhythmically for many times, which is capable of making the center of foot become heated, and at the same time promote the gastrointestinal motility. ③ If the masseur's hands are bigger, three phalangeal joints may be used. ④ For the person who is afraid of itch, for instance, feels an itch as long as the center of foot is touched. At this time, moving manipulation may not be used for the time being.

Indications: Diseases of indigestion and malabsorption, such as abdominal distension, slow empty after eating food.

30. 盲肠和阑尾（图67、68）

定位：位于右脚跟前缘外侧。

手法：示指扣拳法，定点按压3～4次。

辅助手：扶持足背，使其固定，便于主要按摩手顶上力。

注意点：①此点按压时，一是不能移动，二是逐渐用力，目的是既不损伤按摩师的手，又要使对方获得良好的感觉。②也有人用拇指点按的，但示指拳顶法更省力。

适应证：阑尾炎、腹胀、腹泻等。

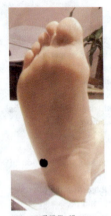

图67 Fig.67

31. 回盲肠（图69红点、70）

定位：右脚跟前外侧的盲肠阑尾反射区前方。

手法：示指扣拳法，定点按压3～4次。

辅助手：同盲肠阑尾的辅手姿势。

注意点：①顶压时，手不要移动。②回盲瓣在医学上是个比较重要的部位。

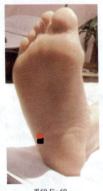

图69 Fig.69

30. Blindgut and appendix (Fig. 67, 68)

Location: In the lateral aspect of the anterior border of the heel of right foot.

Manipulation: Applying buckling manipulation with index finger, the masseur presses the fixed-point for 3-4 times.

Supporting hand: Supporting the dorsum of foot, making it fixed, so as to make it convenient for the main massaging hand to prop with force.

Cautionary notes: ① When pressing this point, do not move and exert force gradually in order to protect the masseur's hand from being injured and make the other side get the good feeling. ② There are still some people who prefer to apply digital-pressing manipulation with the thumb, but the fist propping manipulation with index finger is more labor-saving.

Indications: Appendicitis, abdominal distension, diarrhea, etc.

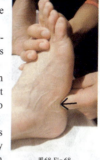
图68 Fig.68

31. ileocecum (the red point in Fig. 69, 70)

Location: Anterior to the reflex zones to blindgut and appendix anterior lateral to the heel of right foot.

Manipulation: Applying hooking fist manipulation with the index finger, press the fixed-point for 3-4 times.

Supporting hand: The same as the posture of the supporting hand for the reflex zones to blindgut and appendix.

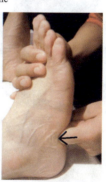
图70 Fig.70

适应证：腹痛、肠炎、便秘、过敏性肠炎、肠梗阻等。

32. 升结肠（图71）

定位：右脚掌外侧，远端达第五跖骨基底内侧端。

手法：以示指扣拳法的示指中节偏桡侧面，由近端向肝区刮压3～4次，逐渐用力并稍停留。

辅助手：握持足背，形成对抗力。

注意点：①此反射区获得适应的感觉有一定难度，一要辅助手对抗用力，二要按摩手用力压入脚掌的情况下向肝区压刮。②为了方便用力，常用力的右手示指压刮，左手辅助。

适应证：急性结肠炎、便秘和腹胀等。

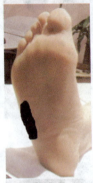

图71 Fig.71

33. 横结肠（图72、73、74）

定位：位于脚步心的脚掌后沿，一般相当于胰和十二指肠的水平线上的横带水平区。

手法：用示指扣拳法的示指中节大面积先压后刮动逐渐加力，3～4次。

辅助手：需在足背用力扶持，固定。

注意点：①右足由外向内，左足由内向外与代谢物在结肠走向一致。②横结肠定位

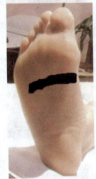

图72 Fig.72

Cautionary notes: ①When propping, do not move the hand. ② Ileocecal valve is a relatively important part in medical science.

Indications: Abdominal pain, enteritis, constipation, enteritis anaphylactica and intestinal obstruction, etc.

32. Ascending colon (Fig. 71)

Location: Lateral to the palm of right foot, with the distal end reaching the medial end of the fifth metatarsal base.

Manipulation: Using the partial radial surface of the middle knuckle of the index finger in the buckling fist manipulation with index finger, the masseur scrapes and presses from medial end to liver zone for 3-4 times, gradually exerting force with slight stay.

Supporting hand: Grip the dorsum of foot, forming counteracting force.

Cautionary notes: ① There is a certain degree of difficulty for this reflex zone to achieve adaptive feeling. Therefore, the counteracting force from the supporting hand is demanded. On the other hand, the massaging hand is required to press and scrape toward the liver zone when forcefully pressing into the palm of foot. ② For the convenience of exerting force, the index finger of right hand is frequently used to press and scrape, with left hand providing help.

Indications: Acute colitis, constipation and abdominal distension, etc.

33. Transverse colon (Fig. 72, 73, 74)

Location: Situated at the posterior border of the palm of foot, through the center of the sole of foot, generally accounting to transverse and horizontal strip area above the horizontal line of pancreas and duodenum.

Supporting hand: It is necessary to support and fix the foot from

应该在胰和十二指肠水平上，不要太靠后。

适应证：急慢性肠炎、结肠炎、腹泻、便秘。

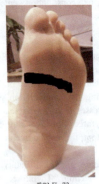

图73 Fig.73

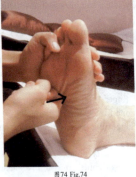

图74 Fig.74

34. 降结肠（图75黑色部分、76）

定位：左脚掌心外侧相当于胰和十二指肠平面至足跟外侧的前方。

手法：用示指压刮法自远而近，逐渐用力，3~4次。

辅助手：左手四个手指尽量在足背外侧用力扒住，便于右手用力压刮。

注意点：两手合力才能压刮出合适的力度，右手示指要直向后刮，到达足跟外前方停住。

适应证：急慢性肠炎、结肠炎、便秘、

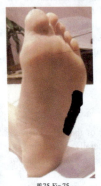

图75 Fig.75

the dorsum of foot.

Manipulation: Use the middle knuckle of index finger in the buckling fist manipulation with index finger to press and then scrape over large area by progressively increasing force for 3-4 times.

Cautionary notes: ① The order is from outside to inside on the right foot, and from inside to outside on the left foot, roughly consistent with the direction in which metabolin travels through colon. ② Transverse colon should be located above the horizontal line of pancreas and duodenum, instead of being located far behind.

34. Descending colon (black part in Fig. 75 and Fig. 76)

Location: Lateral to the center of the palm of left foot, accounting to the area from the plane of pancreas and duodenum to the anterior part of lateral surface of the heel of foot.

Manipulation: Using pressing and scraping manipulation with index finger, press and scrape from distal to local areas by exerting force progressively for 3-4 times.

Supporting hand: With the four fingers of left hand, forcefully hold the foot to the full from the dorsum of foot, so as to forcefully press and scrape with right hand.

Cautionary notes: Combine the two hands so as to press and scrape with proper intensity of force. The index finger of right hand is required to scrape straightly backward and stop when reaching lateral anterior part of heel of foot.

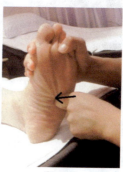

图76 Fig.76

腹胀、消化不良等。

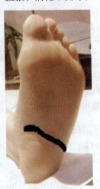

图77 Fig.77

35. 乙状结肠和直肠（图77、78）

定位：自左足跟外前方呈反"S"形移行至右足内前方的膀胱反射区的后方。

手法：用右手示指中节近半部分，从足跟外侧呈反"S"形，先压后扭至足跟的内侧前膀胱反射区后方，3~4次。

辅助手：扶持足背部。

注意点：①右手示指中节压刮时需用腕部和前臂的内旋动作带动。②一定要使示指的关节扭转到膀胱区的后方。

适应证：急慢性结肠炎、肠胃炎、腹胀、腹痛、便秘、腹泻、痔疮等。

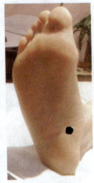

图79 Fig.79

36. 肛门（图79黑点、80）

定位：在足跟部前内方、膀胱后缘的足底和足内侧交界处。

手法：用示指背侧近指间关节顶压，从轻到重逐渐加力，3~4次。

辅助手：扶持足背，使足部固定。

注意点：示指顶压时用力的方向最好从内下向外上方。

适应证：痔疮和其他肛门疾患、肛门括约肌松弛及会阴部其他病症。

Indications: Acute and chronic enteritis, colonitis, constipation, abdominal distension, indigestion, etc.

35. Sigmoid colon and rectum (Fig. 77, 78)

Location: Start from lateral anterior part of heel of left foot, extend in counter-"S" form to the rear of bladder reflex zone at the medial anterior part of right foot.

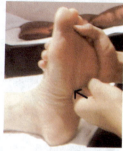

图78 Fig.78

Manipulation: With the proximal half part of the middle knuckle of index finger of right hand, from the lateral surface of heel of foot in counter-"S" form, the masseur presses and then twists to the rear of medial anterior bladder reflex zone of the heel of foot, for 3-4 times.

Supporting hand: Support the dorsum of foot.

Cautionary notes: ① When pressing and scraping with the middle knuckle of right hand, it is necessary to use the inward rotating movements of wrist and forearm bring along. ② Be sure to make the phalangeal joint of index finger twist to the rear of the reflex zone.

Indications: Acute and chronic colitis, enterogastritis, abdominal distension, abdominal pain, constipation, diarrhea, hemorrhoids, etc.

36. Anus (black point in Fig. 79 and Fig. 80)

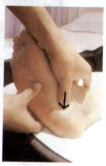

图80 Fig.80

37. 生殖腺（图81、82）

定位：足跟部正中。

手法：用右手示指背侧近指间关节，示指扣拳顶压法顶压，3~4次。

辅助手：扶持并固定足部，也可将辅助的手垫于足跟下，使足跟抬起。

注意点：①顶按时，不要压刮。②根据被按摩者脚的情况，可用按摩棒操作。

适应证：不孕症、性功能低下、失眠、体弱等。

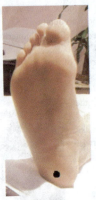

图81 Fig.81

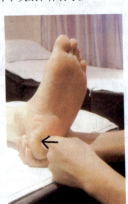

图82 Fig.82

Location: On the anterior medial aspect of heel of foot, at the common boundary of the sole with border of bladder zone and medial surface of foot.

Manipulation: Prop and press with the proximal interphalangeal joint on the dorsal surface of index finger, from light to heavy degree by progressively increasing force, for 3-4 times.

Supporting hand: Support the dorsum of foot, making it fixed.

Cautionary notes: When pressing with the index finger, it is suggestible to exert force in the direction from medial inferior aspect to lateral superior aspect.

Indications: Hemorrhoid and other diseases of anus, anal sphincter dilatation, and other disorders of perineal region.

37. Genital gland (Fig. 81, 82)

Location: Right in the middle of heel of foot.

Manipulation: With the proximal interphalangeal joint on the dorsal surface of index finger, props and presses by applying buckling fist manipulation with the index finger, for 3-4 times.

Supporting hand: Support and fix the foot, or raise the heel of foot by cushioning the heel from below with the auxiliary hand.

Cautionary notes: ① When propping and pressing, do not press and scrape. ② The masseur may operate with the massage stick according to the condition of the massaged.

Indications: Sterility, low sexual function, insomnia, physical weakness, etc.

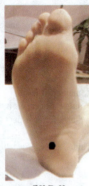

图83 Fig.83

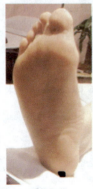

图85 Fig.85

38. 失眠点 (图83黑点、84)

定位：位于生殖腺反射区远侧稍偏内。

手法：同生殖腺手法，用示指扣拳法，顶压3～6次。

辅助手：根据情况，可扶持足背部，也可将足跟部抬高。

注意点：①顶时不可移动。②也可用按摩棒顶压或作横向刮磨。

适应证：失眠、多梦、足跟痛。

39. 腹泻点 (图85黑点、86、87)

定位：足跟与足底交界处后缘正中偏内。

手法：以示指拳顶法，对准足跟与足底交界的后缘偏内处，垂直顶压数次。

辅助手：将足跟抬高并固定。

注意点：①顶压时，示指关节不要移动。②小儿效果较好，但用力要轻，成人用力要重才有效果。

适应证：对于非病源菌引起的腹泻，小儿消化不良效果较佳。

38. Insomnia point (black point in Fig. 83 and Fig. 84)

Location: Situated distally apart from genital gland reflex zone, with slight deviation to medial aspect.

Manipulation: The same as the manipulation of genital gland, i.e., prop and press by applying buckling fist manipulation with the index finger, for 3-6 times.

Supporting hand: According to the detailed situation, support the dorsum of foot or raise the heel of foot.

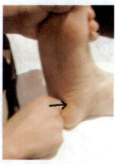

图84 Fig.84

Cautionary notes: ① When propping, one cannot move. ② One can also prop and press with the massage club or scrape and rub transversely.

Indications: Insomnia, dreaminess, talagia.

39. Diarrhea point (black point in Fig. 85 and Fig.86, 87)

Location: Right in the middle of posterior border of the common boundary of heel of foot and sole of foot, with deviation to medial aspect.

Manipulation: Applying fist propping manipulation with index finger, the masseur vertically props and presses for many times by aiming at the partial medial place on the posterior border of the boundary of heel of foot and sole of foot.

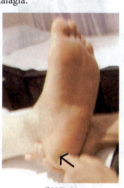

图86 Fig.86

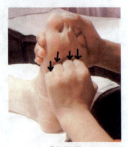

图88 Fig.88

40. 通三焦（图88）

定位：整个足底部。

手法：同推小肠，四指关节直推法。

辅助手：一手固定足背部，不让足左右摆动。

适应证：理气、通调三焦、调节三焦脏腑功能等作用。

（二）足内侧反射区

1. 颈椎（图89、90）

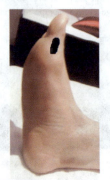

图89 Fig.89

定位：位于踇趾近节趾骨的内侧面。

手法：用拇指端自远至近推3～4次，也可用拇指尖自远至近依次掐捏至第一跖趾关节。

辅助手：扶持并固定脚部。

注意点：①拇指掐捏时要掌握好力度。②也可用示指压刮，或用双指夹持牵拉。

Supporting hand: Highly raise and fix the heel of the foot.

Cautionary notes: ① When propping and pressing, do not move the phalangeal joints of index finger. ② For children, the effect is relatively good, but force should be exerted lightly; for adults, effect can only by achieved by exerting force heavily.

Indications: For diarrhea induced by non-pathogenic bacterium, and child indigestion, good effect can be achieved.

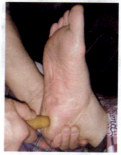
图87 Fig.87

40. Activating triple energizer (Fig. 88)

Location: The whole sole of foot.

Manipulation: The same as the manipulation for pushing the intestine, or straight pushing manipulation with the four finger joints.

Supporting hand: Fix the dorsum of foot with one hand, preventing the foot from swaying from left to right.

Cautionary notes: Regulating qi, activating the triple energizer, regulating functions of the triple energizer and viscera.

Ⅱ. Reflex Zones on Medial Surface of Foot

1. Cervical vertebra (Fig. 89, 90)

Location: Situated at the medial surface of proximal phalanx of thumb toe.

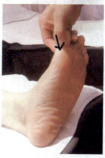
图90 Fig.90

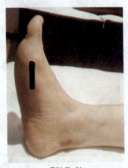

图91 Fig.91

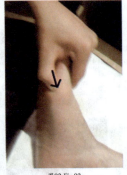

图92 Fig.92

适应证：颈项强硬、酸痛，各种颈椎病以及由颈椎病引起的头、颈、胸、背痛和手部麻痹症等。

2. 胸椎（图91、92）

定位：第一跖骨内侧缘。

手法：用示指压刮法或拇指推法均可，逐次加力并逐渐靠近第一跖骨的骨膜，3～4次。

辅助手：握住足前部或足背部。

注意点：①按摩的力度一定要达到骨膜。②也可用示指钩拳法进行刮磨。③颈椎和胸椎之间是相接的，操作时不要分开。

适应证：胸背部病症，如肩、肩胛骨周围、背部、肋软骨前疼痛、岔气，肋间神经痛，胸痛、胸闷及腹部疾患等。

Manipulation: Use the tip of thumb to push from distal to local areas for 3-4 times, or use the tip of thumb to nip from distal to local areas until reaching the first metatarsophalangeal joint.

Supporting hand: Support and fix the foot.

Cautionary notes: ① Control the intensity of force when nipping with the thumb. ② Or press and scrape with index finger, or drag by clamping with two fingers.

Indications: Stiffness and aching pain of neck, all kinds of cervical spondylopathy, and headache, neck ache, chest ache, backache and paralysis of hand and foot, induced by cervical spondylopathy.

2. Thoracic vertebra (Fig. 91, 92)

Location: The medial border of the first metatarsal bone.

Manipulation: By applying either pressing and scraping manipulation with index finger or pushing manipulation with the thumb, the masseur increases the force progressively and gradually approaches the periosteum of first metatarsal bone, for 3-4 times.

Supporting hand: Grip the anterior part of foot or dorsal part of foot.

Cautionary notes: ① Be sure to make the strength of massage reach the periosteum. ② Or scrape and rub by applying hooking manipulation with index finger. ③ Cervical vertebra and thoracic vertebra are connected with each other, so do not separate the two zones when performing massage.

Indications: Diseases of chest and back, such as shoulder pain, peripheral scapular bone pain, backache, anterior costal cartilage pain, acute pain in chest and rib, intercostal neuralgia, chest pain, chest distress, and abdominal disorders.

3. 腰椎（图93、94）

定位：第一跖骨基底以下，跟骨以前的足弓内侧缘，相当于楔骨和舟骨的内侧部。

手法：与胸椎手法相似，可用示指压刮法，也可用拇指推法，3～4次。

辅助手：握住足前部或足背外侧给予固定。

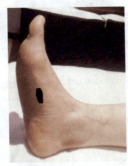

图93 Fig.93

注意点：在腰与骶骨的接合处应用力向上顶。

适应证：腰背痛、腰椎间盘突出症、腰椎后关节紊乱等症。

4. 骶骨（图95、96）

定位：位于脚弓最高处稍后方的跟骨前内侧，前面与腰椎相连。

手法：示指压刮或拇指推法均可，逐渐加力3～4次。

辅助手：按压足内侧前半部固定。

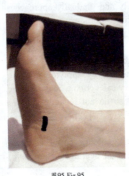

图95 Fig.95

注意点：骶骨反射区在脚弓高处，需用力向上顶压才有效。

3. Lumbar vertebra (Fig. 93, 94)

Location: Medial border of arch of foot, in front of calcaneus, below the base of first metatarsal bone, amounting to the medial part of cuneiform bone and scaphoid bone.

Manipulation: Similar to the manipulation for thoracic vertebra, use either press-scraping manipulation with index finger or pushing manipulation with thumb, for 3-4 times.

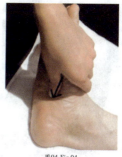

图94 Fig.94

Supporting hand: Fix the foot by gripping the anterior part of foot or the lateral aspect of dorsum of foot.

Cautionary notes: Forcefully prop upward at the conjunction of waist and sacral bone.

Indications: Lumbodorsal pain, lumbar intervertebral disc protrusion, derangement of posterior joint of the lumbar vertebra, etc.

4. Sacrum (Fig. 95, 96)

Location: Situated in the anterior medial aspect of calcaneus, slightly in the rear of the highest place of arch of foot, with the anterior part connected with lumbar vertebra.

Manipulation: Use either the press-scraping manipulation with index finger or pushing manipulation with thumb, progressively increasing the force 3-4 times.

Supporting hand: Fix the foot by

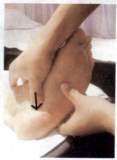

图96 Fig.96

适应证：骶骨部挫伤、骶尾骨脱位、会阴部疾病，如痔疮、大小便异常、前列腺肥大、不孕不育症、性功能低下等。

5. 内尾骨（臀，图97、98）

定位：位于跟骨的后内和下内缘。

手法：用示指钩拳法，分三个动作：①用示指桡侧面钩刮内尾骨的后部。②用示指背侧关节顶着跟骨内下角处。③用示指桡侧面钩刮内尾骨的前下部，反复3遍。

辅助手：垫在足下使足跟部抬高，便于操作。

注意点：以上三个动作要做的扎实。

适应证：骶尾部外伤引起的疼痛、肛门和外阴的疾病、腹泻、大小便失禁、性功能低下等症。

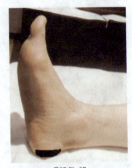

图97 Fig.97

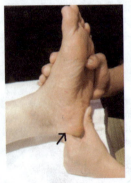

图98 Fig.98

pressing the anterior half of the medial surface of foot.

Cautionary notes: The reflex zone is situated at the top of arch of foot. Therefore the masseur needs to prop upward forcefully to achieve effect.

Indications: Contusion of sacrum, luxation of sacrococcyx, perineal position diseases, such as hemorrhoid, abnormality of urination and defecation, prostatomegaly, infertility and sterility, low sexual function.

5. Internal coccyx (buttocks, Fig. 97, 98)

Location: Situated at posterior medial and inferior medial borders.

Manipulation: Apply hooking manipulation with index finger, which is divided into three movements: ① Hook and scrape the posterior part of the internal coccyx zone with radial surface of index finger. ② Prop the medial inferior corner with the dorsal joint of index finger. ③ Hook and scrape the anterior inferior part of internal coccyx zone with radial surface of index finger, for 3 times repeatedly.

Supporting hand: Make the heel of foot rise by cushioning below the foot, so as to make it convenient to operate.

Cautionary notes: The above three movements should be done thoroughly.

Indications: Pain induced by external injury of sacrococcygeal region, anus and vulva diseases, diarrhea; urinary and fecal incontinence, low sexual function.

6. 子宫或前列腺（图99、100）

定位：足跟内侧，内踝的后下方，呈上小下大的梨子状的区域。

手法：双手拇指推掌法或双拇指扣拳法自下而上压推3~4次，逐渐加力。

辅助手：用双手其余四指固定足部。

注意点：用力先按压再向后上推。

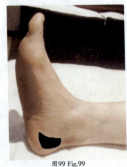
图99 Fig.99

适应证：痛经、子宫病变、尿路感染、前列腺炎、前列腺肥大、性功能低下等。

7. 内肋骨（图101、102）

定位：在足背最高点的后下方凹陷处。

手法：用单拇指扣指法或捏指法均可，逐渐用力3~4次。

辅助手：扶持足部固定。

注意点：①用力扣压时会产生明显放射到肋骨的感觉；②内肋骨周围是胸部，可用拇指推摩。

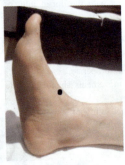
图101 Fig.101

适应证：肋软骨炎、肋软骨损伤、胸闷、岔气、肋间神经痛等症。

6. Uterus or prostate gland (Fig. 99, 100)

Location: On the medial surface of the heel, and the posterior inferior aspect of medial malleolus, the area that takes on pear shape which is big on the top and small at the bottom.

Manipulation: Apply pushing palm manipulation with double thumbs or buckling fist manipulation with double thumbs to press and scrape from top to bottom for 3-4 times, by progressively increasing force.

Supporting hand: Fix the foot with the rest four fingers of the both hands.

Cautionary notes: Forcefully press and then push backward and upward.

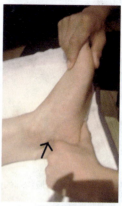

图 100 Fig.100

Indications: Menorrhalgia, metropathia, urinary tract infection, prostatitis, prostatomegaly, low sexual function, etc.

7. Internal rib (Fig. 101, 102)

Location: Situated at the recess, in the posterior and inferior aspect of the highest point on the dorsum.

Manipulation: Applying either buckling manipulation with single thumb or kneading finger manipulation, progressively increase the force for 3-4 times.

Supporting hand: Fix and support the foot.

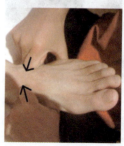

图 102 Fig.102

8. 腹股沟（图103、104）

定位：内踝尖正前方凹陷处。

手法：四个手指置于足底，拇指指腹放于内踝尖处，将指尖顶于伸拇肌腱后方的凹陷内向外侧顶压，每次足背屈内翻时顶压1次，共3次。

辅助手法：握住脚掌部向上内方推，使伸拇肌腱放松。

注意点：①两手配合最重要。②避免压胫骨产生疼痛。

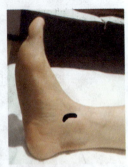

图103 Fig.103

适应证：腹股沟部的疾病、淋巴结炎、疝气、性功能低下、外阴痛症等。

9. 下身淋巴结（图105、106）

定位：内踝前下方的凹陷处。

手法：用拇指尺侧偏峰挤入内踝前下方的凹陷中，取得胀感，反复3～4次。

辅助手：握住足掌部，将足背做跖屈和背屈的运作。

注意点：①当辅助手做跖屈时，按摩手在内踝前下方轻轻挤入。②也可用示指尖代替拇指。

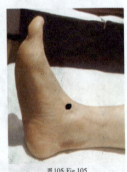

图105 Fig.105

Cautionary notes: ① When the masseur buckles and presses forcefully, the patient will have the obvious feeling that radiates from the zone to the rib. ② The periphery of internal rib zone is the chest zone, to which push-rubbing with thumb may be applied.

Indications: Costal chondritis, injury of costal cartilage; chest distress, acute pain in chest and rib, intercostal neuralgia, etc.

8. Groin (Fig. 103, 104)

Location: At the introcession of just in front of the tip of internal malleolus.

Manipulation: Put the four fingers under the sole of foot, with the finger pulp of thumb placed on the tip of internal malleolus. Prop the finger tip in the introcession in the rear of pollical extensor tendon and then prop and press outward. Every time when dorsiflexion of foot enstrophes, prop and press for once. Altogether there are three times.

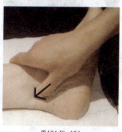

图104 Fig.104

Supporting hand: Grip the palm of foot and push toward the superior and medial aspect, making pollical extensor tendon reflex.

Cautionary notes: ① It is most important for the two hands to cooperate with each other. ② Avoid pressing tibia to cause pain.

Indications: Diseases of groin, lymphnoditis, hernia, low sexual function, vulvodynia, etc.

9. Lymph node in the lower body (Fig. 105, 106)

Location: At the introcession of in the anterior inferior aspect of internal malleolus.

Manipulation: Use the deviation edge of radial surface of thumb to squeeze into the introcession in the anterior-inferior aspect of

适应证：各种炎症、发热、水肿、囊肿、肌瘤、蜂窝织炎、增强抗癌能力以及下肢和会阴处其他病症等。

10. 内侧髋关节（图107、108）

定位：内踝处下和后方的关节缝内。

手法：用拇指捏指法环绕内踝从前下推向下后方的骨缝中，反复3~4次。

辅助手：扶持足背，稍向跖部压，固定之。

注意点：①用拇指捏指或扣指法均可，关键是把力用到内踝距关节缝内，必将出现胀感。②到内踝后方时需用腕部的扭力，拇指尽量往后外推入骨缝。

适应证：髋关节痛、坐骨神经痛、臀大肌损伤等。

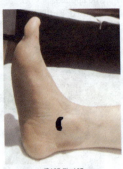

图107 Fig.107

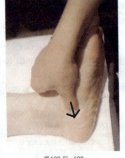

图108 Fig.108

medial malleolus to make the patient get the feeling of distension, for 3-4 times repeatedly.

Supporting hand: Grip the palm of foot and make the dorsum of undergo the movements of foot plantar flexion and dorsal flexion.

Cautionary notes: ① When supporting hand makes the dorsum of foot undergo the movement of foot plantar flexion, the massaging hand lightly squeezes into from the anterior-inferior aspect of internal malleolus. ② Or use index finger to replace the thumb.

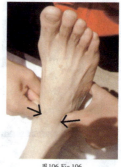

图 106 Fig.106

Indications: All kinds of inflammation, fervescence, hydrops, cystis, muscular tumor, phlegmona, enhancing the ability of anticancer, and other diseases of lower limbs and perineum, etc.

10. Medial coxa joint (Fig. 107, 108)

Location: In the joint suture in the inferior and posterior aspect of internal malleolus.

Manipulation: Applying kneading finger manipulation with thumb, the masseur starts from around internal malleolus and pushes from anterior inferior aspect to inferior posterior aspect of bony suture, for 3-4 times repeatedly.

Supporting hand: Support the dorsum of foot, press slightly towards metarsasus, and fix it.

Cautionary notes: ① Both kneading finger manipulation with thumb or buckling finger manipulation will do. The key point is exert force at internal malleolus and in the joint suture, which is bound to have feeling of turgidity. ② When reaching the rear of

11. 内侧直肠和肛门（图109、110）

定位：胫骨内侧后下方，内踝上3寸以下的带状区，敏感点位于踝后上方。

手法：可用拇指推掌法或示指扣拳法，但要向胫骨的后内缘用力才有感觉。

辅助手：可在足背扶持固定，也可垫于脚下使足跟的后内缘用力才有感觉。

注意点：①该区要想做出感觉来，关键是要刺激到胫骨内踝的后上方。②有时也可用示指钩拳法。

适应证：痔疮、便秘、直肠炎、肛窦炎及腹泻等。

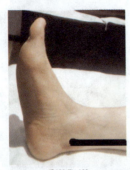

图109 Fig.109

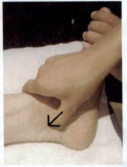

图110 Fig.110

12. 内侧坐骨神经（图111、112）

定位：沿胫骨内后缘上行至胫骨髁下方凹陷为止。

手法：拇指推掌法，由远向近推摩3～5次，逐渐加力。

辅助手：扶持足部，将足背压

internal malleolus, the masseur needs the torsion force from the wrist and push the thumb toward posterior and lateral aspect as much as possible until into the bony suture.

Indications: Coxarthropathy, ischioneuralgia, injury of greatest gluteal muscle, etc.

11. Medial rectum and anus (Fig. 109, 110)

Location: In the posterior inferior aspect of the medial surface of tibia, the strip area below the position 3 Chinese inches above the internal malleolus, with the tenderness point situated in the posterior superior aspect of malleolus.

Manipulation: Apply either pushing palm manipulation with thumb or buckling manipulation with index finger. But the patient can only get the feeling when the masseur exerts force toward the posterior medial border of tibia.

Supporting hand: Support the dorsum of foot, or cushion the foot from below to make the posterior medial border of heel exert force, so as to get feeling.

Cautionary notes: ① To get feeling by performing on the zone, the masseur needs to stimulate the posterior superior aspect of internal malleolus of tibia. ② Sometimes, one can use buckling fist manipulation with index finger.

Indications: Hemorrhoids, constipation, rectitis, anal cryptitis, diarrhea, etc.

12. Medial sciatic nerve (Fig. 111, 112)

Location: Start from medial posterior border of tibia, and go upward until reaching the introcession inferior to condyles of tibia.

Manipulation: Applying pushing palm manipulation with thumb, the masseur push-rubs from distal to local areas 3-5 times, by progressively increasing force.

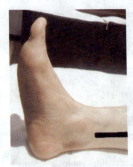

图111 Fig.111

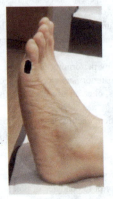

图113 Fig.113

住固定。

注意点：①该区域较长，推之前一定涂好按摩膏。②手法推时要从轻到重逐渐加力，远离胫骨后缘。③在中上1/3交界处注意结节大小与糖尿病的关系，但有结节不一定就有糖尿病。④推动时要缓慢进行。

适应证：坐骨神经痛、坐骨神经炎、糖尿病等。

（三）足外侧反射区

1. 肩（图113、114）

定位：第五跖趾关节为中心。

手法：用示指扣拳法分外、前、后三个方向自远而近各压刮3~4次。

辅助手：各方向手法分别辅助，压刮外侧时，辅助手虎口顶住足内侧第一跖趾关节处；压刮前侧先用拇指顶住第五跖趾关节下方；压刮后侧先用中、示指扒住第五跖趾关节背后部。

Supporting hand: Support the foot and fix the dorsum of foot by pressing it.

Cautionary notes: ① The area is a little bit longer, so be sure to apply massage ointment before pushing. ② When using pushing manipulation, one should gradually increase the force keeping away from posterior border of tibia. ③ Pay attention to the size of nodus in relation to diabetes at the juncture 1/3 the distance in middle upper position, but nodus does not necessarily mean diabetes. ④ Perform slowly when pushing.

Indications: Ischioneuralgia, ischiatitis, diabetes, etc.

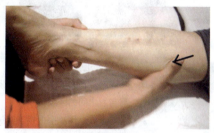

图112 Fig.112

III. Reflex Zone in Lateral Aspect of Foot

1. Shoulder (Fig. 113, 114)

Location: Centering around the fifth metatarsophalangeal joint.

Manipulation: Apply buckling fist manipulation with index finger to press and scrape in the lateral, anterior and posterior directions from distal to local areas for 3-4 times repectively.

Supporting hand: Provide help for the manipulation in different directions respectively. When the masseur presses and scrapes the lateral aspect, he should prop against the first metatarsophalangeal joint in the medial aspect of foot with hukou of the supporting hand.

注意点：①两手配合很重要。②脚掌有脚垫时，可用定点顶压肩后侧。

适应证：肩周炎、手臂麻木无力等。

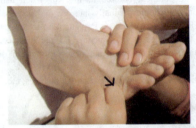

图114 Fig.114

2. 上臂（图115、116）

定位：第五跖骨外面和上面，在肩与肘之间的区域。

手法：用单手拇指推掌法或示中两指压刮法自远而近从轻逐次重推3～4次。

辅助手：因用双手拇指推法，无需辅助。

注意点：用双手拇指推掌法利于该处的血液循环，被按摩者也感到舒服。

适应证：治疗上肢的各种不适症。

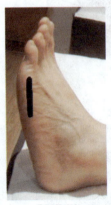

图115 Fig.115

When the masseur scrapes the anterior aspect, he should prop against the inferior aspect of the fifth metatarsophalangeal joint with the thumb of the supporting hand. When masseur presses and scrapes the posterior aspect, he should hold the dorsal posterior aspect of first metatarsophalangeal joint with the middle and index fingers of the supporting hand.

Cautionary notes: ① It is important for the two hands to cooperate with each other. ② When there is foot pad on the palm of foot, one may prop and press the posterior aspect of shoulder with fixed point.

Indications: Periarthritis of shoulder, numbness and weakness of arm, etc.

2. Upper arm (Fig. 115, 116)

Location: On the lateral and superior surfaces of fifth metatarsal bone, the area between the shoulder and elbow.

Manipulation: Apply pushing palm manipulation with single thumb or pressing and scraping manipulation with index and middle fingers to push from far to near side with gradually increasing force for 3-4 times.

Supporting hand: There is no need to provide help, for using pushing palm manipulation with double thumbs.

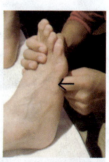

图116 Fig.116

Cautionary notes: Using pushing palm manipulation with double thumbs is beneficial to the blood circulation of the area, and meanwhile, the massaged feels comfortable.

Indications: All kinds of discomforts of upper limbs.

3. 肘（图117、118）

定位：第五跖骨基底部前后外侧的凹陷处。

手法：用示指扣拳法分别按压第五跖骨基底外侧前后两个凹陷处。也可用示中两指关节同时顶压这两个凹陷。

辅助手：扶持并顶住足内侧。

注意点：①操作前一定要先摸清第五跖骨基底的两个凹陷。②分别按压的方法好些。

适应证：网球肘、肱骨内上髁炎、肘关节外伤和其他原因引起的上肢痛。

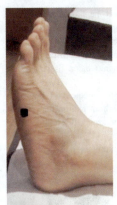

图117 Fig.117

4. 膝（图119、120）

定位：脚外侧外踝下方的凹陷处。

手法：单示指扣拳法，自前向后旋扭180°，在前、上、后三处各点压一次，从轻到重做3~4次。

辅助手：扶持足踝部固定。

注意点：①膝关节有两种做法：一种是从前向后一直旋扭180°，这种方法敏感度高，止痛效果好。还有一种是从前点开始。扭、点、扭、点，

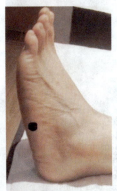

图119 Fig.119

3. Elbow (Fig. 117, 118)

Location: At introcessions anterior posterior lateral to the basal part of the fifth metatarsal bone.

Manipulation: By using buckling fist manipulation, the masseur presses the anterior and posterior introcessions lateral to the base of the fifth metatarsal bone respectively, or the masseur may use the two interphalangeal joints in the middle of index finger to prop-press the two introcessions simultaneously.

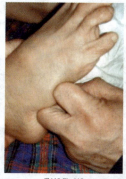

图118 Fig.118

Supporting hand: Support and prop the medial aspect of foot.

Cautionary notes: ① Before operation, be sure to grope for the two introcessions of the base of the fifth metatarsal bone at first. ② The method of pressing respectively is better.

Indications: Tennis elbow, medial humeral epicondylitis, trauma of elbow joint, and the upper limb pain induced by other reasons.

4. Knee (Fig. 119, 120)

Location: At the introcession inferior to the lateral malleolus on the lateral surface of foot.

Manipulation: By using buckling fist manipulation with single index finger, the masseur rotates from front to rear for 180°, and digital-presses once in anterior, superior and posterior positions respectively, with gradually increasing force 3-4 times.

Supporting hand: Support and fix the ankle.

Cautionary notes: ① There are two methods for dealing with knee joint: one is to rotate from front to rear up to 180°, which is of

每90°点一下。此法较温和。②该反射区对老年人特别重要。

适应证：膝关节各部的伤痛、炎症和老年性膝关节增生引起的疼痛等。

5. 外尾骨（图121、122）

定位：足跟外下和外后方。

手法：用示指钩拳法从足跟后上方跟腱止点开始钩刮足跟外侧的后下交界处时，改用示指关节直顶法，再变成示指钩拳法完成外下方的钩刮，反复3~4次。

辅助手：将足跟垫高。

注意点：对足跟部比较粗糙者可用按摩棒压刮。

适应证：骶尾部外伤和臀部挫伤引起的疼痛、臀肌损伤和臀外侧皮神经损伤等。

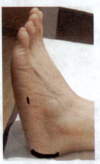

图121 Fig.121

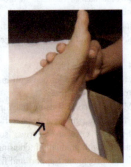

图122 Fig.122

high tenderness and good effect of alleviating pain. The other is to begin with digital-pressing from front, and then, rotate, digital-press, rotate, digital-press, with one digital-pressing every 90°. This method is relatively gentle. ② The reflex zone is of vital importance to aged people.

Indications: Traumatic pain in different parts of knee joint, inflammation, and the pain induced by senile proliferation of knee joint, etc.

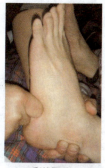

图120 Fig.120

5. External coccyx (Fig. 121, 122)

Location: Lateral-inferior to and lateral-posterior to the heel of foot.

Manipulation: Apply hooking manipulation with the index finger, and start from the ending point of Achilles tendon posterior superior to the heel of foot. When beginning to hook and scrape the posterior-inferior juncture lateral to the heel of foot, the masseur changes to use straight propping manipulation with the joint of index finger, and then change to use hooking manipulation with index finger to finish the hooking and scraping of lateral inferior aspect, for 3-4 times repeatedly.

Supporting hand: Cushion the heel of foot higher.

Cautionary notes: For the patient with relatively rough heel of foot, the masseur use massage stick to scrape-press.

Indications: Pains induced by injury of sacrococcyx and contusion of buttock, injury of gluteal muscles and injury of lateral cutaneous nerve of the buttock.

6. 外侧生殖腺（图123、124）

定位：足跟部外侧，踝关节后下方，呈上小下大的梨子形状的区域。

手法：用示指钩拳法，从轻逐次加力，由上后至下前方钩刮3~4次。

辅助手：将手垫于足下方，使其抬高或扶持足跖内侧以固定之。

注意点：①不要用力太大，避免疼痛。②注意用力的方向。③与足底生殖腺同属一反射区。

适应证：不孕症、性功能低下、失眠、体弱等症。

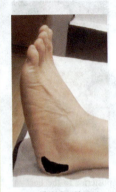

图123 Fig.123

7. 肩胛骨（图125、126）

定位：足背第四、第五跖骨与楔骨间呈一带状区域。

手法：双拇指推掌法，由远至近逐渐加力推向楔骨骨突处，左右分开，推7~8次。

辅助手：因双手同时操作，不需固定。

注意点：①此区较长，又在足背，故手法要轻。②用指腹推，不要用指尖推。

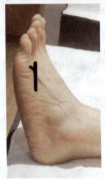

图125 Fig.125

6. Lateral genital gland (Fig. 123, 124)

Location: Lateral to the heel of foot, and posterior inferior to ankle joint, the area that takes on the pear shape which is small at top and big at bottom.

Manipulation: Using hooking manipulation with the index finger, and progressively increasing the force from light degree, the masseur hook-scrapes from superior posterior aspect, to inferior anterior aspect, for 3-4 times.

Supporting hand: Cushion under the foot with hand, raising the foot higher or fix the foot by supporting the inferior aspect of the sole of foot.

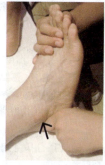

图124 Fig.124

Cautionary notes: ① Do not exert too strong force, so as to avoid pain. ② Pay attention to the direction of exerting force. ③ This zone belongs to the same reflex one as that of genital gland on the sole of foot.

Indications: Infertility, low sexual function, insomnia, and debility.

7. Scapula (Fig. 125, 126)

Location: A strip area between the fourth and fifth metatarsal bones and cuneiform bone.

Manipulation: Applying pushing palm manipulation with double thumbs, the masseur pushes toward the catapophysis of the cuneiform bone by progressively increasing force from far to near end. Separating left from right, the masseur

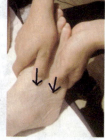

图126 Fig.126

适应证：肩背后酸痛、肩周炎、肩关节外伤、肩活动受限等。

8. 外肋骨（图127、128）

定位：第三、第四楔骨凹陷处，表面有一定软包块鼓起，第五跖骨粗隆内后方。

手法：用拇指指端捏指法或用示指关节点揉法，从轻缓慢捏3次。

辅助手：用两手拇指顶住足底，两手指关节同时按压内外两个反射区。

注意点：①此处血管丰富而脆，不宜用大力扣点。②最好用左手捏揉左足，右手捏揉右足。

适应证：各种肋间神经痛、胸闷、胸膜炎、肩周炎、肩胛骨酸痛、肩痛、腰背痛等。

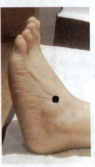

图127 Fig.127

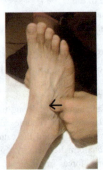

图128 Fig.128

pushes 7-8 times.

Supporting hand: There is no need to fix the foot for the two hands are involved in operation simultaneously.

Cautionary notes: ①This reflex zone longer and is situated at dorsum of foot, so light manipulation is needed. ② Push with the finger pulp in stead of the fingertip.

Indications: Aching pain of the dorsal surface of the shoulder, scapulohumeral periarthritis, trauma of shoulder joint, limitation of shoulder motion, etc.

8. Lateral rib (Fig. 127, 128)

Location: At the introcession of the third and fourth cuneiform bones, with a certain heave like soft lump on the surface, medial posterior to the tuberosity of the fifth metatarsal bone.

Manipulation: Using nipping finger manipulation with the tip of the thumb or digital-kneading manipulation with the phalangeal joint of index finger, the masseur slowly nips from light degree for 3 times.

Supporting hand: Prop the sole of foot with the two thumbs, with the phalangeal joints of the two hands pressing medial and lateral reflex zones.

Cautionary notes: ① The blood vessels here are plentiful and fragile. It is not appropriate to use strong force to press the point. ② It is suggestible to use left hand to nip-knead the left foot, and right hand for the right foot.

Indications: All kinds of intercostal neuralgia, chest distress, pleuritis, scapulohumeral periarthritis, aching pain of scapula, shoulder pain, lumbago, etc.

9. 上身淋巴结（图129、130）

定位：外踝前下方的凹陷中。

手法：同上反射区手法，待足背伸时趁机挤入，反复3～4次。

辅助手：握持足前部做背伸和背屈动作。

注意点：①先用拇指或示指轻轻触摸该区的骨缝。②最好用拇指虎口侧偏峰，也可用指尖。

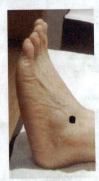

图129 Fig.129

10. 外侧髋关节（图131、132）

定位：外踝内侧的前方、下方和后方的骨缝。

手法：拇指扣推外踝前下后方的骨缝，逐渐加力3～4次。出现胀感为度。

辅助手：扶持足背向内侧和跖部施压。

注意点：①将力送入外踝内方的骨缝中，取得胀感是关键。②注意推至下后方时，需扭动腕关节，将拇指桡侧峰尽量挤入骨缝中。

适应证：髋关节外伤、臀上皮神经炎、臀部及下肢部其他病痛等。

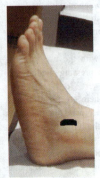

图131 Fig.131

9. Lymph node in the upper body (Fig. 129, 130)

Location: In the introcession anterior inferior to lateral malleous.

Manipulation: The same as the manipulation for the above reflex zone. Take the opportunity to squeeze into the introcession when the dorsum of foot extends, repeatedly for 3-4 times.

Supporting hand: Grip the anterior part of foot, making dorsal extention and flexion.

Cautionary notes: ① First of all, lightly touch the bony suture of the reflex zone with the thumb and the index finger. ② Use the lateral deviation edge of hukou, or use the fingertip.

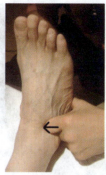

图 130 Fig.130

10. Lateral coxa joint (Fig. 131, 132)

Location: The bony suture anterior to, superior posterior to the medial aspect of lateral malleolus.

Manipulation: Buckle-push the bony suture anterior–superior–posterior to the medial aspect of lateral malleolus, and progressively increase force for 3-4 times, until the patient get feeling of distension.

Supporting hand: Support the dorsum of foot and press toward the medial aspect and metatarsus.

Cautionary notes: ① Exert the force into the bony suture medial to the medial

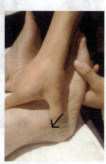

图 132 Fig.132

11. 下腹部 （图133）

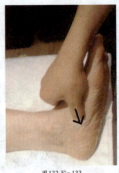

图133 Fig.133

定位：外踝后方的凹陷带状区，上界不超过外踝上四横指。敏感点位于外踝后上方。

手法：用拇指推掌法或示指钩拳法均可，做3~4次。

辅助手：扶持足背固定或将手放于足跟下，将此反射区抬高。

注意点：示指钩拳法易做出敏感点。

12. 外侧坐骨神经 （图134、135）

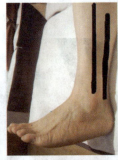

图134 Fig.134

定位：小腿外侧的腓骨后方的长形区域和胫骨与腓骨之间的胫前肌均定为外侧坐骨神经反射区。

手法：用拳推法。逐渐加力3~4次。

辅助手：扶持足背，固定小腿。

注意点：①必须紧握拳头。②必须先压后推，并一直保持均匀压力，3~4次。

适应证：腿腰疼痛、坐骨神经痛、下肢关节痛及小腿和足部的疲劳等。

aspect of the lateral malleolus. The key point is to get the feeling of distension. ② Attention should be paid to twist the wrist when pushing the inferior posterior aspect, and make the radial surface of the thumb squeeze into the bony suture as much as possible.

Indications: Trauma of hip joint, superior clunial neuritis, and other diseases of the buttock and lower limbs, etc.

11. Lower abdominal part (Fig. 133)

Location: The depressed strip area posterior to the lateral malleolus, the upper bound of which does not exceed the range of four fingers above the lateral malleolus. The tenderness point is situated at the place posterior-superior to the lateral malleolus.

Manipulation: Both the pushing palm manipulation with the thumb and the hooking fist manipulation with the index finger will do. Perform for 3-4 times.

Supporting hand: Fix the foot by supporting the dorsum of foot, or put the hand under the heel of foot, raising this reflex zone higher.

Cautionary notes: It is easy to produce the tenderness point by using the hooking fist manipulation with the index finger.

12. Lateral sciatic nerve (Fig. 134, 135)

Location: The long area posterior to the fibula lateral to the shank, and the anterior tibial muscle between the tibia and fibula are both called lateral sciatic nerve reflex zone.

The tenderness point is situated at the place posterior-superior to the lateral malleolus.

Manipulation: Apply pushing palm

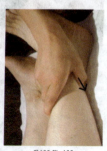

图 135 Fig.135

（四）足背反射区

1. 上鄂（上颌，图136、137）

定位：足𧿹趾趾间关节的远侧。

手法：拇指推掌扣指法，由内向外连续推摩3~4次，逐次加力。

辅助手：以拇、示指将足𧿹趾末节捏住并向下压弯，使𧿹趾趾间关节屈曲，背侧暴露清楚。

注意点：①按摩时的拇指只向外推，不要来回推扒。②要靠紧关节线推摩。③如欲增加美容效果，可加用拇指端扣捏甲根和甲旁的部位。

适应证：牙痛、面部美容、口腔及口腔的各种病症。

2. 下鄂（下颌，图136、137）

定位：足𧿹趾趾间关节的近侧。

手法：同上反射区用拇指推掌法、扣指法，由内向外连续推摩3~4次。

辅助手：以拇、示指将足𧿹趾末节捏住并向下压弯，使𧿹趾弯曲，背侧关节暴露明显。

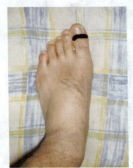

图136 Fig.136

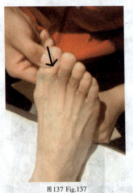

图137 Fig.137

manipulation, and progressively increase force for 3-4 times.

注意点：①辅助手不要只捏甲部再向下弯造成不适。②按摩时只向外推，不要来回推摩。③要靠紧关节线推摩。

适应证：牙痛、面部美容、口腔溃疡、鼻腔和舌部的疾患等。

3. 扁桃腺（图138、139）

定位：足蹞趾近节趾骨背侧中段两旁。

手法：用两拇指指端或示指关节同时扣压趾近节背部中段两侧，3～4次。

辅助手：因双手操作，只好用两手的示、中指在蹞趾后方固定蹞趾了。

注意点：①定位要准，确实扣捏在蹞趾近节背侧中段两侧。②用力角度斜向上方。

适应证：感冒、扁桃体炎、咽炎、鼻炎、喉炎等。

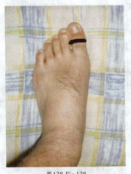

图138 Fig.138

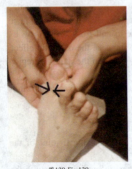

图139 Fig.139

thumb and the buckling finger manipulation for the above reflex zone. Continuously push-rub from inside to outside for 3-4 times.

Supporting hand: Nip the paratelum of the big toe with the thumb and index finger and bend it downward, making the interphalangeal joint of the big toe flex and the dorsal surface exposed clearly.

Cautionary notes: ①The supporting hand is not allowed to bend the big toe by nipping the nail only, which will bring about indisposition. ② When massaging, only push outward instead of pushing and rubing to and fro. ③ Push-rub by adhering to the joint line.

Indications: Toothache, facial beauty, dental ulcer, and diseases of nasal cavity and tongue.

3. Tonsil (Fig. 138, 139)

Location: Two sides of intermediate segment of dorsal surface of proximal phalanx of the big toe.

Manipulation: Buckle-press with the fingertips of the two thumbs or the interphalangeal joints of the index fingers two sides of intermidiate segment of dorsal surface of proximal phalanx of the big toe, for 3-4 times.

Supporting hand: Because the two hands are involved in the operation, the masseur can only fix the big toe from behind it with the index and middle fingers of the two hands.

Cautionary notes: ① Make accurate location and secure buckle-nipping two sides of intermediate segment of dorsal surface of proximal phalanx of the big toe. ② Exert the force obliquely upwards.

Indications: Common cold, tonsillitis, pharyngitis, rhinitis, laryngitis, etc.

4. 咽喉（图140、141）

定位：第一跖趾关节外上方的骨突起处。敏感点偏背侧稍远点。

手法：用示指推掌法先触到第一跖趾关节外侧的骨突，再扣向趾背侧，则出现明显的胀感，按压3～4次。

辅助手：扶持足背外侧，使其固定。

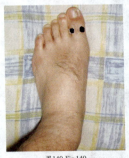
图140 Fig.140

注意点：①操作要领是先摸到第一跖趾关节外侧的骨突，再向趾背侧扣敏感点；②有明显症状者，可增加扣捏次数。

适应证：咽炎、鼻炎、扁桃体炎、声音嘶哑、吞咽异常和其他上呼吸道感染等症。

5. 胸部淋巴腺（图142、143）

定位：在第一跖骨的外侧缘。

手法：同上述手法用示指推掌法，一边扣捏第一跖骨外侧缘，一边向内侧用力推向近端，第一跖骨底，反复3～4次。

辅助手：扶持固定足部外侧。

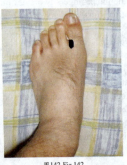
图142 Fig.142

注意点：①胸部淋巴腺也叫胸腺，是个重要的免疫器官，尤其对

4. Throat (Fig. 140, 141)

Location: Catapophysis superior to the first metatarsophalangeal joint, with the tenderness point deviated slightly far from the dorsal surface.

Manipulation: Using pushing palm manipulation, the masseur first touches the catapophysis lateral to the first metatarsophalangeal joint, and then buckles the dorsal surface of the toe, and the patient will feel obvious distending. Press for 3-4 times.

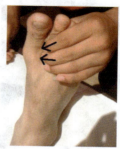

图141 Fig.141

Supporting hand: Fix the dorsum of foot by supporting the lateral surface of it.

Cautionary notes: ① The essentials of operation are: first touch the catapophysis lateral to the first metatarsophalangeal joint, and then buckle the tenderness point toward the dorsal surface of the toe. ②For the patient with overt symptom, one may increase the number of times of buckle-nipping.

Indications: Pharyngitis, rhinitis, tonsillitis, hoarse voice, abnormality of deglutation, and other diseases of upper respiratory tract infection.

5. Thoracic lymph gland (Fig. 142, 143)

Location: At the lateral border of first metatarsal bone.

Manipulation: Apply pushing palm manipulation with the index finger, which is the same as the above mentioned manipulation. While buckle-nipping the lateral border of first metatarsal bone, the masseur pushes toward the proximal end, base of first metatarsal bone by exerting force toward the medial aspect, repeatedly for 3-4 times.

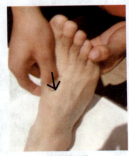

图143 Fig.143

婴儿更为重要。②在操作时，一定要注意沿第一跖骨外侧向内用力推，才能出现麻胀的感觉。③推至第一跖骨基底部的外侧。

适应证：各种炎症、胸痛、癌症和一切提高免疫能力的疾病。

6. 气管（图144、145）

定位：位于第一跖骨基底外侧。

手法：同上述手法用单示指推掌法，向第一跖骨基底的内后方用力，取得酸胀痛感，反复3~4次。

辅助手：扶持足前部外侧。

注意点：①此点是气管反射区，也是气管的敏感点。②每次在推完胸腺后，顺势向内后顶压气管敏感点，使其出现胀痛感。

适应证：咽干、声嘶、咳嗽、哮喘、急性气管炎等。

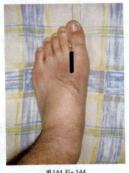

图144 Fig.144

Supporting hand: Support and fix the lateral surface of foot.

Cautionary notes: ① Thoracic lymph gland is also called thoracic gland, which is an important immune organ, especially more significant for infants and children. ② When operating, be sure to push forcefully inwards along the lateral surface of first metatarsal bone, so as to get the feeling of numbness and turgidness. ③ Push to the lateral aspect of the base of first metatarsal bone.

Indications: Various kinds of inflammation, chest pain, cancer, and all the diseases that need to deal with by enhancing immune competence.

6. Trachea (Fig. 144, 145)

Location: Situated at the lateral surface of base of the first metatarsal bone.

Manipulation: Apply pushing palm manipulation with the index finger, which is the same as the above mentioned manipulation. While buckle-nipping the lateral border of first metatarsal bone, the masseur pushes toward the proximal end, base of first metatarsal bone by exerting force toward the medial aspect, repeatedly for 3-4 times.

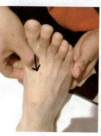

图145 Fig.145

Supporting hand: Support and fix the lateral surface of foot.

Cautionary notes: ① The point is a sensitive point of the trachea. ② Apply pushing palm manipulation with the single index finger, which is the same as the above mentioned manipulation. Exert force toward the medial posterior aspect of the first metatarsal bone so as to get the feeling of sourness, turgidness and pain.

Indications: Dry pharynx, hoarseness, cough, asthma, acute tracheitis, etc.

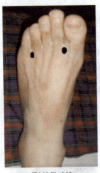

图146 Fig.146

7. 内耳（图146、147）

定位：足背第一、第二跖骨及第四、第五跖骨关节间。

手法：用两示指推掌法，由远至近，沿第五跖趾关节内沿向后推，逐次加力，3~4次。

辅助手：扶持足掌的内侧。

注意点：耳鸣、耳聋、头晕、眼花、晕车、晕船、血压低、梅尼埃综合征等。

8. 胸部和乳房（图148、149）

定位：位于第二、第三、第四跖骨足背侧形成的大片状区域。

手法：双拇指推掌法，从轻渐重，多次推摩，面积要大，推3~5次。

辅助手：双手操作无需辅助。

注意点：推摩次数不限，对于失眠、疲劳和围绝经期综合征的患者可以增加至数十次。

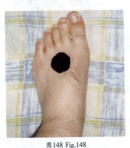

图148 Fig.148

适应证：胸闷、胸痛、乳腺炎、乳腺增生、生产乳汁不足、乳腺癌、失眠、围绝经期综合征等。

7. Inner ear (Fig. 146, 147)

Location: Between the interphalangeal joints of first and second metatarsal bone, and between the interphalangeal joints of fourth and fifth metatarsal bone.

Manipulation: Using pushing palm manipulation, from far to near side, the masseur push backward along the medial aspect of the metatarsophalangeal joint, by progressively increasing the force, for 3-4 times.

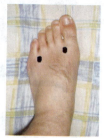

图147 Fig.147

Supporting hand: Support the medial aspect of the palm of foot.

Cautionary notes: Apply pushing palm manipulation with the single index finger, which is the same as the above mentioned manipulation. Exert force toward the medial posterior aspect of the first metatarsal bone, so as to get the feeling of sourness, turgidness and pain, repeatedly for 3-4 times.

Indications: Tinnitus, deafness, dizziness, dim eyesight, car-sickness, train-sickness, and sea-sickness, low blood pressure, Meniere's syndrome, etc.

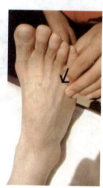

图149 Fig.149

8. Chest and breast (Fig. 148, 149)

Location: Situated at large lamellar area formed by the dorsum of the first, second and third metatarsal bones.

Manipulation: Applying pushing palm manipulation with the two thumbs, from light to heavy degree, the masseur push-rubs for

9. 膈肌（图150、151）

定位：经过足背部最高点的横形带状区。一般相当于跖跗关节处。

手法：用双示指钩拳法，由足背中央开始刮到足背两侧到足底交界处，3～6次。

辅助手：双手拇指抵住足掌部以助力。

注意点：①开始时用力均匀舒适。②要由最高点的中央开始。

适应证：胸闷、胸痛、呃逆、恶心、腹部和胸胁不适等。

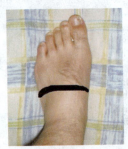

图150 Fig.150

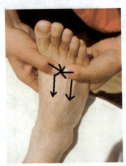

图151 Fig.151

10. 输卵管或输精管（图152、153）

定位：内侧连于内踝后下方的前列腺（或子宫），外侧与足背外侧的睾丸（或卵巢）相接，中间经过内外踝前方的胫距关节线，形成一条横向带状区。

手法：用双手示指钩拳法从中央向两侧钩摩到内外跟骨侧面，逐渐加力3～6次。

辅助手：同膈肌反射区的操作辅助法。

注意点：①该区操作时注意不要压痛内外踝；②尽量延长到

several times, covering larger range. Push like that for 3-4 times.

Supporting hand: There is no need of supporting, for both hands are involved in operation.

Cautionary notes: There is limit of the number of push-rubbing. For the patient with insomnia, fatigue, climacteric syndrome, one may increase tens of times.

Indications: Chest distress, chest pain, mammitis, hyperplasia of mammary gland, insufficient lactation; breast cancer, insomnia, climacteric syndrome, etc.

9. Diaphragmatic muscle (Fig. 150, 151)

Location: The horizontal strip area across the highest point on top of the dorsum of foot, generally amounting to the tarsometatarsal joint.

Manipulation: Using hooking fist manipulation with double index fingers, the masseur scrapes from the center of the dorsum of foot to the two sides of the dorsum of foot to the juncture of the sole of foot, for 3-6 times.

Supporting hand: Prop the palm of foot with the double thumbs, so as to provide assistance.

Cautionary notes: ① Exert force evenly and comfortably at the beginning. ② Start from the center of the highest point.

Indications: chest distress, chest pain, pseudoglottic myoclonia, nausea, indisposition of abdomen and chest and hypochondrium, etc.

10. Oviduct and deferent duct (Fig. 152, 153)

Location: The medial aspect connected with the prostate gland (or uterus) posterior inferior to internal malleolus, the lateral aspect connected with the testicles lateral to the dorsum of foot, the intermedial aspect traversing the tibial astragaloid joint line anterior to the medial and lateral malleolus, and forming a horizontal strip area.

内外足跟侧面。

适应证：附件炎、输卵管阻塞、不孕症、前列腺炎和性功能低下等。

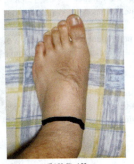

图152 Fig.152

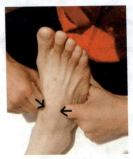

图153 Fig.153

11. 上、下身淋巴结（图154、155）

定位：上身淋巴结位于外踝前下方的凹陷处；下身淋巴结位于内踝前下方的凹陷中。

手法：同上法用双手示指钩拳法，用示指节桡侧突起部轻轻挤压，得酸胀感时，反复按压3~4次。

辅助手：同上。

注意点：①定位要准，手法

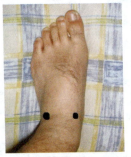

图154 Fig.154

Manipulation: Using hooking fist manipulation with double index fingers, the masseur hook-rubs from the center to the two sides to the lateral aspects of medial and lateral heel bones, by progressively increasing the force for 3-6 times.

Supporting hand: The same as the auxilary operation for diaphragmatic muscle.

Cautionary notes. ① When operating at the zone, pay attention not to press the medial and lateral malleolus to the point of feeling pain. ② Extend to the lateral surfaces of the medial and lateral heel bones as far as possible.

Indications: Appendagitis, impatency of oviduct, infertility, prostatitis, low sexual function, etc.

11. Lymph node in upper and lower body (Fig. 154, 155)

Location: Lymph node in upper body is situated at the introcession anterior inferior to lateral malleolus; lymph node in lower body situated at the introcession anterior inferior to medial malleolus.

Manipulation: Using hooking fist manipulation with double index fingers the same as the above, the masseur lightly squeeze-presses with

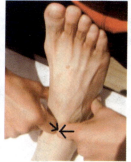

图155 Fig.155

the enation of the radial surface of the phalangeal joint of the index finger, untill getting the feeling of sourness and tugidness. Repeatedly press for 3-4 times.

Supporting hand: The same as above.

Cautionary notes: ① make accurate location, and the manipualtion requires progressively increasing force. ② It is required for the patient

要由轻到重逐渐加力。②要有酸胀感。

适应证：各种炎症、发热、水肿、足踝痛和免疫力低下引起的病症。

12. 解溪（图156、157）

定位：位于足背两踝关节前横纹中点，两筋之间。

手法：用一手拇指尖扣入解溪中，另一手旋扭踝关节获得胀感，按压3~5次。

辅助手：握住足部，顺时针和逆时针旋转扭踝关节。

注意点：①辅助手做扭踝时要缓慢，要逐步达到最大角度。②解溪是全身最后一个反射区，以上操作结束后一定要再重复足底的排泄系统的按摩。

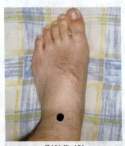

图156 Fig.156

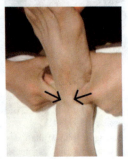

图157 Fig.157

to get the sensation of soreness and distension.

Indications: Various kinds of inflammation, fever, dropsy, ankle pain, and the diseases induced by hypoimmunity.

12. Jiexi (Fig. 156, 157)

Location: Situated between the middle point of anterior transverse striation of the two ankle-joints and the two tendons.

Manipulation: The masseur buckles into the Jiexi with one thumb, and rotates the ankle-joint with the other hand, until the patient gets the feeling of tugidness. Press for 3-5 times.

Supporting hand: Grip the foot, and clockwise and anti-clockwise rotate the ankle-joint.

Cautionary notes: ① The supporting hand should be slowly when rotating the ankle, gradually up to the maximum angle. ② Jiexi is the last reflex zone in the whole body, do repeat the massage of excretory system on the sole of foot after the above operation is finished.

最后做整理手法：如屈伸踝关节、搓揉足背、足心，拍击足底等如图158~161。

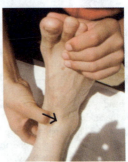

图158 Fig.158

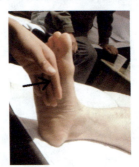

图159 Fig.159

Rearrange the manipulation: Extend and flex the joint, knead the dorsum of foot, planter center, flap the sole of foot, as shown in Fig. 158-161.

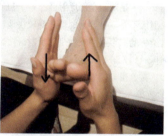

图160 Fig.160

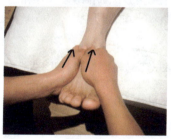

图161 Fig.161

第四章 双足整体按摩

前面我们介绍了足部的全部反射区,对于初学者来说,要很快记牢这些反射区不是一件容易的事,要较快地牢记各反射区的定位必须经常给你的同事或朋友做足部反射区按摩,才能掌握足部的常用反射区。

足部反射区按摩讲究要有一定的顺序,凡是按顺序按摩的都能起到良好的效果。但在实际操作过程中,又要把握"全部按摩,重点突出"的观点,这也是取得良好效果的保证。对于慢性病来说,一方面调整了全身的功能,另一方面促进了有病器官的恢复。对于急性病来说,因时间较紧,更要重点突出,只需做主要的几个反射区。下面介绍几个重点的反射区。

第一节 基本反射区

"肾、输尿管、膀胱"这三个反射区为基本反射区,因为它们代表排泄系统。促进排泄系统的功能,把体内有毒物质和酸性产物随尿液排出体外是防治一切疾病和调整全身各器官生理功能不可缺少的步骤,因此把它称为"基本反射区"。

第二节 直接反射区

有病痛对应足部的同名或异名同功的反射区叫病症反射区,也叫直接反射区。无论病症性质如何,都要这样选区。这是配区的第二步骤。如胃痛,无论是胃炎,还是胃痉挛,都要选取胃反

Chapter 4 Integral Massage of Two Feet

In previous part, we have introduced the whole reflex zones on the foot. It is not easy for beginners to bear in mind all these reflex zones. To quickly keep in mind the location of each reflex zone, you must frequently perform massage on foot reflex zones for your colleagues or friends, so as to grasp the commonly used reflex zones on the foot.

Foot reflex zone requires a certain order. Anyone who performs massage in proper order can achieve favourable result. In actual operation, however, one needs to stick to the principle of "Massaging all over and focusing on the key point", which guarantees the achievement of favourable effect. For chronic diseases, the massage helps to regulate the function of the whole body and promote the recovery of the organ with disorder. For acute diseases, one should further focus on the key point, that is, massage on several main reflex zones, for the time is relatively urgent. Some key reflex zones are introduced as follows.

Section 1 Basic Reflex Zones

The three reflex zones of "kidney, ureter, bladder" are basic reflex zones, for they represent excretory system. Promoting the function of excretory system and expelling toxic substance and acid products out of body along with urine are the indispensable steps for the prevetion and treatment of all diseases, and regulation of physiological function of organs in the whole body. Hence, they are called "basic reflex zones".

Section 2 Direct Reflex Zones

There are some diseases that correspond to the reflex zones on

射区；再如眼部疾病，无论是近视，还是青光眼、白内障，都要选用眼反射区。

第三节 相关反射区

疾病形成是复杂的，有病器官从许多方面与其他器官和系统发生不同程度的联系。因此，选择与病症器官和系统相关的反射区是个较复杂的问题。需要从不同的角度考虑。这也是配区的第三步骤。主要根据以下三点进行选择：

根据西医解剖结构：从西医解剖关系选配反射区，包括相邻关系、支配关系或协同关系等。如头痛选额窦、三叉神经、小脑和脑干颈椎等。

根据中医脏腑辨证、五行相生原则：五行间按木（肝）生火（心），火生土（脾），土生金（肺），金生水（肾），水生木的次序，生者为母，被生者为子。按"虚者补其母，实者泻其子"的原则，某脏发生病变时，如为虚证，则在补该脏的同时，还要补其母脏；再如某脏为实证时，则要泻其子脏，肝火实证，在泻肝火的同时，还要泻心火，即按摩心脏反射区以达到泻的作用。

the foot with the same or different names but the same functions, we call these reflex zones illness reflex zones, or direct reflex zones. One must choose the reflex zone like that regardless of the nature of the illness. This is the second step for allocation of zones. Take stomach ache for instance, one should choose stomach reflex zone no matter whether it is gastritis or gastrospasm; Take ocular disease for another example, one should choose eye reflex zone no matter whether it is glaucoma or cataract.

Section 3 Correlated Reflex Zones

It is very complicated for the formation of diseases. The organ with disease tends to correlate at different levels with other organs or systems. Therefore, it is relatively complicated to choose the reflex zone that correlates with the affected organ and system. One needs to take it into consideration from different angles. This is also the third step for the allocation of zones. One may choose mainly in accordance with the following three points:

In line with anatomic structure of western medicine:

Choose and allocate the reflex zones from the anatomic relations of Western medicine, including neighbouring, dominating, or coordinating relations. For headache, one may choose frontal sinus, trigeminal nerves, cerebellum, brain stem, cervical vetebra, etc.

In the light of TCM principles of syndrome differentiation according to viscera, and generation among five elements:

The five elements correlate with each other by following the sequence of wood (liver) generating fire (heart), fire generating earth (spleen), earth generating metal (lung), metal generating water (kidney), and water generating earth. The generator is called the mother organ, while the generated is called the child organ. Hence, there is a principle called "tonifying the mother organ in case of deficiency and reducing the child organ in case of excess". When

根据疾病性质：

1. 感染性疾病应着重刺激与提高人体抵抗力有关的反射区，如脾、上下身淋巴结、胸部淋巴结等。

2. 慢性消耗性疾病患者在选配反射区时应加消化系统反射区。

3. 过敏性疾病应重点选用肾上腺和甲状旁腺反射区等。

4. 内分泌疾病，如糖尿病、月经不调，应加强内分泌系统反射区，再加其他相关反射区。

第四节 配区结合原则

下面介绍的是部分常见病的配区原则及按摩组合，在应用时尤其要多体会主要的敏感点。

【各系统所含反射区】

首先要了解人体的十大系统：神经系统、呼吸系统、循环系统、消化系统、泌尿系统、生殖系统、内分泌系统、免疫系统、感觉系统以及运动系统。十大系统与反射区存在以下对应关系：

1. 排泄系统（基本反射区）：包括肾、输尿管、膀胱和尿道等。

2. 神经系统：大脑、小脑、脑干、三叉神经、脊柱、腹腔神经丛等。

3. 呼吸系统：鼻、咽喉、气管、支气管、肺、横膈膜、胸部等。

4. 循环系统：包括心脏、肺、上身淋巴结、下身淋巴结等。

pathological change occurs in a certain organ, one should tonify the organ, meanwhile reinforcing its mother organ, if it belongs to asthenia syndrome; and one should purge the organ, meanwhile reducing its mother organ, if it belongs to sthenia syndrome. Take sthenia syndrome of hepatic fire for example, when purging the hepatic fire, one has to reduce the cardiac fire. That is, one should massage the heart reflex zone so as to achieve purging effect.

According to the nature of diseases:

1. For infectious diseases, one should focus on simulating the reflex zones that are interrelated with the improvement of power of resistance of human body, such as spleen, lymph nodes in upper and lower body, thoracic lymph node, etc.

2. For the patient with chronic wasting disease, one should add the reflex zones to digestive system when choosing and allocating reflex zones.

3. For anaphylactic disease, one should focus on choosing reflex zones to adrenal gland and parathyroid gland, etc.

4. For endocrine diseases, such as diabetes, irregular menstruation, one should add reflex zones to endocrine system and other related reflex zones.

Section 4 The Principles of Allocation and Combination of Reflex Zones

Principles of allocation of reflex zones and massage combination for some common diseases are introduced as follows. One should especially attach importance to the comprehension of main tenderness points.

The reflex zones contained in the systems

First of all, one needs to get to know the ten systems of human body: nervous system, respiratory system, circulatiory system, digestive system, urinary system, genital system, endocrine system,

5. 消化系统：上下颚、食管、胃、十二指肠、小肠、盲肠、阑尾、升结肠、降结肠等。

6. 生殖系统：男性前列腺、输精管、睾丸、阴茎、腹股沟、下腹部；女性：子宫、输卵管、卵巢、阴道、腹股沟、下腹部等。

7. 内分泌系统：脑垂体、肾上腺、甲状腺、甲状旁腺、胰脏等。

8. 免疫系统：脾、胸腺、上身淋巴结、上下身淋巴结、扁桃体等。

9. 运动系统：脊柱、斜方肌、肩甲骨、肩、肘、膝、髋、内外肋骨、内外坐骨神经等。

10. 感觉系统：眼、耳、内耳、鼻等反射区。

【常见病配区举例】

(一) 神经系统疾病

1. 失眠：排泄系统、内分泌系统和消化系统等。

2. 头痛：排泄系统、头颈部、腹腔神经丛、肝、胆内分泌和免疫系统等。

3. 精神紧张：排泄系统、神经、消化系统和内分泌等。

4. 中风：排泄、神经、循环、内分泌、消化和运动系统等。

5. 植物神经功能紊乱：排泄、神经、内分泌、消化和免疫系统等。

6. 记忆力减退：排泄、神经、内分泌、消化和免疫系统等。

immune system, sensory system and motor system. There exist the following corresponding relations between the ten systems and the reflex zones.

1. Excretory system (basic reflex zones): including kidney, ureter, bladder, urethra, etc.

2. Nervous system: cerebrum, cerebellum, brain stem, trigeminal nerves, spinal column, coelial plexus, etc.

3. Respiratory system: nose, throat, trachea, bronchus, lung, diaphragm, chest, etc.

4. Circulatory system: heart, lung, lymph node in upper body, lymph node in lower body, etc.

5. Digestive system: upper and lower jaws, esophagus, stomach, duodenum, small intestine, blindgut and appendix, ascending colon, decending colon, etc.

6. Genital system: male: prostate gland, deferent duct, testicle, penis, groin, lower abdomen, etc; female: uterus, oviduct, ovary, vagina, groin, lower abdomen, etc.

7. Endocrine system: hypophysis, adrenal gland, thyroid gland, parathyroid gland, pancreas, etc.

8. Immune system: spleen, thoracic gland, lymph node in upper body, lymph node in lower body, tonsilla, etc.

9. Motor system: spinal column, trapezius muscle, scapula, shoulder, elbow, knee, coxa joint, interior and exterior ribs, interior and exterior sciatic nerves, etc.

10. Sensory system: eye, ear, inner ear, nose, etc.

Examples of allocation of zones for common diseases

Ⅰ. Nervous system diseases

1. Insomnia: excretory, endocrine and digestive, system etc.
2. Headache: excretory system, head and neck, coelial plexus, liver, gall, endocrine and immune systems, etc.

(二) 五官科疾病

1. 结膜炎：排泄系统、头颈部、消化系统等。

2. 屈光不正：排泄系统、头颈部、循环系统、内分泌系统和消化系统等。

3. 干眼症：排泄系统、头颈部、循环系统、内分泌系统和肝胆等。

4. 中耳炎：头颈部、排泄系统、内分泌系统和免疫系统等。

5. 过敏性鼻炎：排泄系统、头颈部、呼吸系统、内分泌系统和肝胆等。

6. 副鼻窦炎：排泄系统、头颈部、呼吸、内分泌和免疫系统等。

7. 咽喉炎：排泄系统、呼吸系统、颈项、颈椎和免疫系统等。

(三) 呼吸系统疾病

1. 感冒：排泄系统、头颈部、呼吸、内分泌和免疫系统等。

2. 哮喘：排泄系统、颈椎、胸部和乳房、呼吸、内分泌、免疫和消化系统等。

3. 肺气肿：排泄、呼吸、循环、内分泌、免疫、消化系统和胸椎等。

(四) 循环系统疾病

1. 心前痛：排泄、循环、颈椎、胸椎、内肋骨、肩胛骨、胸部和乳房、呼吸、内分泌、胃十二指肠、消化腺等。

2. 冠心病：排泄、循环、呼吸、消化、内分泌和免疫系统以及脊柱等。

3. Mental strain: excretory, nervous, digestive, and endocrine systems, etc.

4. Apoplexy: excretory, nervous, circulation, endocrine, digestive, locomotor systems, etc.

5. Functional disorder of vegetative nerve: excretory, nervous, endocrine, digestive and immune systems, etc.

6. Decrescence of the faculty of memory: excretory, nervous, endocrine, digestive and immune systems, etc.

Ⅱ. Diseases of five senses

1. Conjunctivitis: excretory system, head and neck, and digestive systems, etc.

2. Refractive errors: excretory system, head and neck, circulatory, endocrine, and digestive system.

3. Xeroma: excretory system, head and neck, circulatory, endocrine system, and liver and gall, etc.

4. Tympanitis: head and neck, endocrine, endocrine, and immune system, etc.

5. Allergic rhinitis: excretory system, head and neck, respiratory system, endocrine system, and liver and gall, etc.

6. Paranasal sinusitis: excretory system, head and neck, respiratory, endocrine, and immune system, etc.

7. Sphagitis: excretory, respiratory system, neck and nape, cervical vertebra, and immune systems, etc.

Ⅲ. Diseases of respiratory system

1. Common cold: excretory system, head and neck, respiratory, endocrine, and immune system, etc.

2. Asthma: excretory system, cervical vertebra, chest and breast, respiratory system, endocrine system, immune system, and digestive system, etc.

3. Emphysema: excretory, respiratory, circulatory, endocrine, immune, and digestive systems and thoracic vertebra, etc.

3. 心率不齐：神经、循环、呼吸、内分泌系统等。

4. 高血压：排泄、循环、内分泌、运动和生殖系统等。

5. 下肢怕冷：排泄、循环、内分泌、运动和生殖系统等。

（五）消化系统疾病

1. 厌食症：排泄、神经、消化、内分泌、免疫和运动系统等。

2. 消化不良：排泄、消化、内分泌系统等。

3. 急性胃肠炎：排泄、消化、内分泌、免疫、神经、呼吸和循环系统等。

4. 牙痛：上下颚、头颈部等。

5. 牙龈炎：排泄、神经、消化和内分泌系统等。

6. 胃炎：排泄、神经、消化、内分泌和免疫系统等。

7. 十二指肠溃疡：排泄、消化、循环、神经、内分泌和免疫系统等。

8. 腹胀：排泄、消化、神经和内分泌系统等。

9. 胆石症：排泄、消化、内分泌和循环系统等。

10. 糖尿病：排泄、消化、内分泌、循环、免疫及内外侧坐骨神经等。

11. 便秘：排泄、消化、生殖、循环、消化和免疫系统等。

12. 痔疮：排泄、消化、生殖和骶尾骨等。

（六）泌尿系统疾病

1. 肾炎：排泄、生殖、神经、内分泌和免疫系统等。

2. 膀胱炎：排泄、生殖、神经、内分泌和免疫系统等。

3. 排尿困难：排泄、生殖、神经、内分泌、免疫和运动等。

IV. Diseases of circulatory systems

1. Precordialgia: excretory, circulatory system, cervical vertebra, thoracic vertebra, internal rib, scapula, chest and breast, respiratory, endocrine system, stomach, duodenum, digestive gland, etc.

2. Coronary artery disease: excretory, circulatory, respiratory, digestive, endocrine, immune systems and spinal column, etc.

3. Irregularity of heart rate: nervous, circulatory, respiratory, endocrine systems, etc.

4. Hypertension: excretory, circulatory, endocrine, motor, and genital systems, etc.

5. Lower limbs dreading cold: excretory, circulatory endocrine, motor, and genital systems, etc.

V. Diseases of digestive system

1. Apositia: excretory, nervous, digestive, endocrine, immune, motor systems, etc.

2. Indigestion: excretory, digestive, endocrine systems, etc.

3. Acute gastroenteritis: excretory, digestive, endocrine, immune, nervous, respiratory, circulatory systems, etc.

4. Toothache: upper and lower jaws, head and neck, etc.

5. Gingivitis: excretory, nervous, digestive, and endocrine, etc.

6. Gastritis: excretory, nervous, digestive, endocrine, and immune system, etc.

7. Duodenal ulcer: excretory, digestive, circulatory, nervous, endocrine, and immune systems, etc.

8. Abdominal distension: excretory, digestive, nervous, and endocrine systems, etc.

9. Cholelithiasis: excretory, digestive, endocrine, and circulatory systems, etc.

10. Diabetes: excretory, digestive, endocrine, and circulatory, immune systems, and medial and lateral sciatic nerves, etc.

11. Constipation: excretory, digestive, genital, circulatory, and

4. 尿失禁：排泄、生殖、神经、运动、内分泌和免疫系统等。

(七) 生殖系统疾病

1. 前列腺炎：排泄、生殖、神经、内分泌和免疫系统等。
2. 子宫肌瘤：排泄、生殖、内分泌、免疫和神经系统等。
3. 子宫内膜炎：排泄、生殖、内分泌和免疫系统等。
4. 盆腔炎：排泄、生殖、神经、循环、消化、内分泌、免疫和运动等。
5. 缺乳：排泄、神经、呼吸、循环、消化、生殖和内分泌系统等。
6. 月经不调：排泄、生殖、神经、循环、消化和内分泌系统等。

(八) 内分泌系统疾病

1. 甲状腺功能亢进和功能低下：排泄、神经、内分泌、消化和循环系统等。
2. 肥胖症：排泄、神经、内分泌、循环、消化、运动和免疫系统等。
3. 骨质疏松：排泄、神经、内分泌、循环、消化、运动和免疫系统等。
4. 儿童发育不良：排泄、神经、内分泌、消化、运动和生殖系统等。
5. 围绝经期综合征：排泄、神经、循环、内分泌、消化和生殖系统等。

immune systems, etc.

12. Haemorrhoids: excretory, digestive, genital systems, and sacrococcyx, etc.

Ⅵ. Diseases of urinary system

1. Nephritis: excretory, genital, nervous, endocrine, and immune systems, etc.

2. Cystitis: excretory, genital, nervous, endocrine, and immune systems, etc.

3. Dysuresia: excretory, genital, nervous, endocrine, immune, and motor systems, etc.

4. Urinary incontinence: excretory, genital, nervous, motor, endocrine, and immune systems, etc.

Ⅶ. Diseases of genital system

1. Prostatitis: excretory, genital, nervous, endocrine, and immune systems, etc.

2. Hysteromyoma: excretory, genital, endocrine, immune, and nervous systems, etc.

3. Endometritis: excretory, genital, endocrine, and immune systems, etc.

4. Pelvic inflammation: excretory, genital, nervous, circulatory, digestive, endocrine, immune, and motor systems, etc.

5. Lack of lactation: excretory, nervous, respiratory, circulatory, digestive, genital, and endocrine systems, etc.

6. Irregular menstruation: excretory, genital, nervous, circulatory, digestive, endocrine systems, etc.

Ⅷ. Diseases of endocrine system

1. Hyperthyroidism and hypothyroidism: excretory, nervous, endocrine, digestive, and circulatory systems, etc.

2. Obesity: excretory, nervous, endocrine, circulatory, digestive, motor, and immune systems, etc.

(九) 免疫系统疾病

1. 过敏性疾病：排泄、内分泌、免疫、消化和神经系统等。
2. 脾肿大：排泄、内分泌、免疫、消化和内分泌系统等。

(十) 运动系统疾病

1. 颈椎病：排泄、头颈部、运动、呼吸和循环系统等。
2. 背痛：排泄、头颈部、脊柱、呼吸、循环和消化系统等。
3. 腰痛：排泄、运动、神经、生殖、内分泌、循环和消化系统等。
4. 肩周炎：排泄系统、运动系统、头颈部。
5. 岔气：神经系统、呼吸系统等。
6. 膝关节痛：脊柱、运动系统等。
7. 膝关节肿痛：排泄、运动、神经、内分泌、免疫和生殖系统等。
8. 下肢酸痛：排泄、运动、循环、消化和内分泌系统等。
9. 风湿和类风湿关节炎：排泄、神经、呼吸、循环、消化、运动、内分泌和免疫系统等。

3. Osteoporosis: excretory, nervous, endocrine, circulatory, digestive, motor, and immune systems, etc.

4. Childhood maldevelopment: excretory, nervous, endocrine, digestive, motor, and genital systems, etc.

5. Climacteric syndrome: excretory, nervous, circulatory, endocrine, digestive and genital systems, etc.

IX. Disease of immune system

1. Anaphylactic disease: excretory, endocrine, immune, digestive, and nervous systems, etc.

2. Enlarged spleen: excretory, endocrine, immune, digestive, and nervous systems, etc.

X. Diseases of motor disease

1. Cervical syndrome: excretory system, head and neck, motor, respiratory, and circulatory systems, etc.

2. Dorsalgia: excretory system, head and neck, spinal column, respiratory, circulatory, and digestive systems, etc.

3. Lumbago: excretory, motor, nervous, genital, endocrine, circulatory, and digestive systems, etc.

4. Scapulohumeral periarthritis: excretory, motor systems, and head and neck, etc.

5. Acute pain in chest and rib: nervous and respiratory systems, etc.

6. Knee-joint pain: spinal column, motor system, etc.

7. Knee-joint swelling and pain: excretory, motor, nervous, endocrine, immune, and genital systems, etc.

8. Aching pain in the lower limbs: excretory, motor, circulatory, digestive, and endocrine systems, etc.

9. Rheumatic and rheumatoid arthritis: excretory, nervous, respiratory, circulatory, digestive, motor, endocrine, and immune systems, etc.

（十一）皮肤病

1. 荨麻疹：排泄、神经、内分泌、免疫和消化系统等。
2. 面部痤疮：排泄、头颈部、内分泌、免疫、生殖和呼吸系统等。
3. 湿疹：排泄、神经、内分泌、消化和免疫系统等。
4. 斑秃和脱发：排泄、神经、内分泌、免疫和消化系统等。
5. 带状疱疹：排泄、神经、消化、内分泌和免疫系统等。

（十二）其他症状

1. 疲倦：排泄、神经、运动、循环、消化、内分泌和免疫系统等。
2. 醉酒：排泄、神经、呼吸、消化和内分泌系统等。
3. 身体虚弱：排泄、神经、循环、消化、内分泌和免疫系统等。
4. 浮肿：排泄、循环、消化、内分泌和运动系统等。
5. 晕厥：排泄、头颈部、内分泌系统等。

XI. Dermatogic diseases

1. Urticaria: excretory, nervous, endocrine, immune, and digestive systems, etc.

2. Facial acne: excretory system, head and neck, endocrine, immune, genital, and respiratory systems, etc.

3. Eczema: excretory, nervous, endocrine, digestive, and immune systems, etc.

4. Alopecia areata and defluvium capillorum: excretory, nervous, endocrine, immune, and digestive systems, etc.

5. Acute posterior ganglionitis: excretory, nervous, digestive, endocrine, and immune systems, etc.

XII. Other symptoms

1. Languor: excretory, nervous, motor, circulatory, digestive, endocrine, and immune systems, etc.

2. Drunkenness: excretory, nervous, respiratory, digestive, and endocrine systems, etc.

3. Debilitation of body: excretory, nervous, circulatory, digestive, endocrine, and immune systems, etc.

4. Puffiness: excretory, circulatory, digestive, endocrine and motor systems, etc.

5. Apopsychia: excretory, head and neck, and endocrine systems, etc.